The Essential Handbook of Healthcare Simulation

Healthcare simulation is the modern way to educate healthcare providers to achieve high performance and improve patient safety. It encompasses mannikin-based training for practicing teamwork and nontechnical skills in the context of a clinical case, task trainers for procedural skills, simulated participants for communication skills, and virtual/augmented reality simulation.

This text is founded on experience gained through establishing an accredited centre for excellence in healthcare simulation – the Irish Centre for Applied Patient Safety and Simulation (ICAPSS) and its associated award-winning postgraduate course. This essential handbook provides the background knowledge required to run a healthcare simulation centre; use simulation for training and education; and support simulation-based quality improvement and research activities.

Paul O'Connor, PhD, MA, MSc, BSc (Hons), Personal Professor, School of Medicine, University of Galway, and Research Director, Irish Centre for Applied Patient Safety and Simulation.

Angela O'Dea, PhD, MSc, MSc, BA, HDip, Senior Lecturer in Patients Safety, Human Factors, and Simulation, Irish Centre for Applied Patient Safety and Simulation, University of Galway.

Dara Byrne, MB BCh BAO, MScEd, MCh, FRCSI, Clinician and Professor of Simulation, University of Galway, and Director of the Irish Centre for Applied Patient Safety and Simulation.

The Essential Handbook of Healthcare Simulation

Paul O'Connor

Angela O'Dea

Dara Byrne

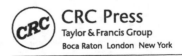

CRC Press

Taylor & Francis Group

Boca Raton London New York

CRC Press is an imprint of the
Taylor & Francis Group, an **informa** business

First edition published 2024
by CRC Press
6000 Broken Sound Parkway NW, Suite 300, Boca Raton, FL 33487-2742

and by CRC Press
4 Park Square, Milton Park, Abingdon, Oxon, OX14 4RN

CRC Press is an imprint of Taylor & Francis Group, LLC

ISBN: 978-1-032-28467-5 (hbk)
ISBN: 978-1-032-27993-0 (pbk)
ISBN: 978-1-003-29694-2 (ebk)

DOI: 10.1201/9781003296942

Typeset in Times
by SPi Technologies India Pvt Ltd (Straive)

Contents

Chapter 1 Introduction, History, and Key Concepts 1

Introduction 1
Purpose of This Book 2
Chapter Outline 2
Ethical Imperative of Simulation-based Education 2
Types of Healthcare Simulators 3
    Manikin Simulators 3
    Simulated Participants 4
    Task Trainer/Part-Task Trainer 4
    Computer-based Simulators 5
    Virtual Reality Simulators 5
    Table-top Simulation 5
Sim Zones 6
Simulation and Realism 6
Effectiveness of Simulation 7
Healthcare Simulation Societies and Conferences 8
Healthcare Simulation Journals 9
Conclusion 9
Further Reading 9
Online Resources 10
References 10

Chapter 2 Learning Theories 12

Introduction 12
Chapter Outline 12
Adult Learning Theory 13
Behavioural Learning Theory 13
    Deliberate Practice 14
    Precision Teaching 15
    Task Analysis 16
Social Cognitive Learning Theory 16
Constructivist Learning Theory 18
    Experiential Learning 18
Combining Different Learning Theories 19
    Simulation-based Mastery Learning 20
Conclusion 21
Further Reading 21
References 21

Chapter 3 Instructional Design 23

Introduction 23
Chapter Outline 23
The ADDIE Model 23
Stage 1: Analyse 24

Stage 2: Design..26
    Learning Outcomes and Learning Objectives 26
    Teaching Strategy 27
Stage 3: Develop...28
Stage 4: Implement...29
Stage 5: Evaluate 30
    New World Kirkpatrick Model 32
    Training Evaluation Designs 33
Final thoughts on the ADDIE Model 35
Conclusion...35
Further Reading...35
Online Resources...36
References 36

Chapter 4   Scenario Writing..38

Introduction 38
Chapter Outline 38
Scenario Writing 38
Writing Team Simulation Scenarios...39
    Title...39
    Case Summary..39
    Scene Information 40
    Faculty Information 40
    Initial Patient Information 40
    Further Patient Information 41
    Supporting Team or Faculty 41
    Technical/Environmental Requirements...42
    Scenario States, Learner Actions and Triggers...............................43
    Further Considerations for Writing Team Scenarios 43
Writing Simulated Participant Scenarios 43
    Overview and Administrative Details..44
    Notes and Learner Instructions..44
    Case Content for SPs 45
    Further Considerations for Writing SP Scenarios 46
Conclusion...46
Further Reading...46
References 46

Chapter 5   Physical Safety in Simulation...47

Introduction 47
Chapter Outline 47
Physical Safety of Simulation 47
Risks to Patients 48
    In Situ Simulation – Purpose and Efficacy.....................................48
    Risk of Interference with Real Patient Care 48
    Risk Associated with the Use of Medication....................................49
    Risks Associated with the Use of Simulated and Real Medical Devices
    and Medical Equipment...51

Risks Associated with Patient Records..51
Risk of Inappropriate Use of Hospital Resources 52
Risk of Negative Transfer...52
Risks to Learners..52
Risks to Simulated Participants..53
Risks to Simulation Facility Staff...53
Developing a Simulation Facility Safety Policy..................................53
Form a Steering Group for Development and Implementation of the
Simulation Safety Policy 54
Identify Existing Safety Procedures for the Health Service/Educational
Institution That Are Relevant for the Simulation Facility 54
Incorporate Existing Simulation Safety Practices 54
Consider the Hazards and Extent of Predicted Safety Risk On the
Literature and Local Experience 54
Prioritise Medication Safety and Liaise with Pharmacy
Representatives..55
Effectively Communicate the Existence of the Simulation Safety Policy,
and the Need for Staff Involved in Simulation Delivery to
Comply 55
Enable Simulation Faculty to Conduct Safe Simulation Sessions That
Are Compliant with the Policy 55
Develop a Reporting Process for Simulation-Related Adverse Events Or
Near-misses, Preferably Integrated Within the Health Services' Clinical
Adverse Event Reporting Framework 55
Conclusion...56
Further Reading...56
Online Resources...56
References 56

Chapter 6   Psychological Safety and Prebriefing..57

Introduction 57
Chapter Outline 57
Psychological Safety 57
Threat to Professional Identify 58
Threat of Validity...58
Threat of Hidden Agendas...58
Threats Associated with Particular Types of Scenarios 58
Scenarios That Utilise Deception 58
Death of the Simulator Scenarios 59
Equality, diversity, and inclusion (EDI) Scenarios...........................60
Threat to the Psychological Safety of Simulated Participants...........60
Establishing a Safe Learning Environment 61
Prebriefing 62
Describing What the Learners Can Expect during the
SBE Activity 62
Describing What Is Expected of the Learners 63
Conclusions 64
Further Reading...65
Online Resources...65
References 65

Chapter 7   Debriefing..67

    Introduction 67
    Chapter Outline 67
    What Is Debriefing?...68
        Reflection...68
        Debriefing and the Experiential Learning Cycle 68
    Psychological Safety and Debriefing 68
    Debriefing Strategies 69
        Strategy 1: Address the Learning Objectives..69
        Strategy 2: Structure the Debriefing 70
        Strategy 3: Select an Appropriate Conversational Strategy 71
        Strategy 4: Select the Appropriate Time Point for the Debrief.................72
        Strategy 5: Utilise Skilled Facilitators...72
        Strategy 6: Consider if Video-Assisted Debriefing (VAD) Is Appropriate......73
        Strategy 7: Consider Using Standardised or Scripted Debriefing 74
    Debriefing as Formative Assessment..74
    Difficult Debriefing Situations 75
    Faculty Training and Development 76
        Debriefing the Debrief..76
        The Observational Structured Assessment of Debriefing Tool (OSAD) 76
        Debriefing Assessment for Simulation in Healthcare (DASH) 77
    Conclusion...78
    Further Reading..78
    Online Resources...79
    References 79

Chapter 8   Assessment...81

    Introduction 81
    Chapter Overview..82
    Assessment 82
        Formative and Summative Assessment 82
        Objective Structured Clinical Examination (OSCE) 83
    Determining the Usefulness of Assessment 83
        Reliability 83
        Validity 84
        Feasibility 84
        Educational Impact...85
    Assessment Frameworks 85
        Assessing Procedural Skills..85
        Assessing Non-technical Skills 86
    Assessing Simulation Educators 89
    Conclusion...90
    Further Reading..90
    Online Resources...90
    References 90

Chapter 9   Running a Simulation Facility...92

    Introduction 92
    Chapter Outline 92
    Simulation Facility Priority Areas..93

Priority Area 1: Governance Structure 93
    Leadership 93
    Mission and Vision Statements 94
    Steering Committee 94
Priority Area 2: Programme Management 94
    Instructional Design 94
    Policies and Procedures 94
Priority Area 3: Resource Management 95
    Financing 95
    Selecting and Purchasing Equipment 95
    Inventorying Equipment 96
    Storage of Equipment 96
    Facilities 96
Priority Area 4: Personnel 96
    Staffing 97
    Job Descriptions 97
Priority Area 5: Faculty and Staff Development 97
    Education, Training, and Qualifications 97
    Staff Accreditation or Certification 98
Priority Area 6: Programme Assessment 98
    Evaluation   98
    Learner Feedback 98
    Faculty Evaluation 98
    Simulation Management Systems 99
    Facility Accreditation 99
Priority Area 7: Integrity 99
    Adoption of a Code of Ethics 99
Priority Area 8: Promoting the Activities of a Simulation Facility 99
    Local Promotion 100
    Website and Social Media 100
    National and International Promotional Activities 100
Simulation Facility Strategic Planning 100
Conclusions 101
Further Reading 101
Online Resources 102
References 102

Chapter 10 Using Simulation for Research 104

Introduction 104
Chapter Overview 104
Types of Simulation Research 104
    Research about Simulation 105
    Research through Simulation 105
Conducting Simulation Research 106
Writing a Simulation Research Publication 107
    Title and Abstract 108
    Introduction 108
    Method 109
    Results 109
    Discussion 109
    Authorship 110

Choosing Where to Publish Simulation Research..111
Submitting Your Manuscript...111
Responding to Reviewer Comments 112
Other Forums for Sharing Simulation Research 112
Conclusion...112
Further Reading...113
Online Resources...113
References 113

Chapter 11 The Use of Simulation for Quality Improvement..................................115
Introduction 115
Chapter Overview..115
QI and Research 115
Use of Translational Simulation for QI 116
Simulation for Diagnosis..116
    Individual Factors 117
    Team Factors..117
    Technology Factors...118
    Work Environment Factors...120
    Systems Factors 120
    Simulation for Adverse Event Investigation...121
Simulation for Improvement 122
Reporting QI Studies...123
Conclusion...124
Further Reading...124
References 124

Appendix 1 Team Scenario Development Template...126
Appendix 2 Standardised Participant Case Development Template 145
Index..158

1 Introduction, History, and Key Concepts

KEY POINTS

- Healthcare simulation consists of any tool, device, and/or environment that mimics an aspect of clinical care.
- Simulation has been used to educate and train healthcare providers for thousands of years.
- Simulation-based education provides an approach for addressing the ethical tension of the need for healthcare providers to learn, and the delivery of safe patient care.
- There are a wide range of different healthcare simulators available – each with different strengths and weaknesses.
- Increased realism in simulation does not necessarily translate to better learning outcomes.
- Care should be taken in using impact on clinical outcomes as a measure of the effectiveness of simulation-based education.
- There are many simulation societies, conferences, and journals to support new, and existing, simulationists.

INTRODUCTION

Healthcare simulation consists of any tool, device, and/or environment that mimics an aspect of clinical care, and which shares a broad, similar purpose – to improve the safety and effectiveness of healthcare services (Cook et al., 2011; Levine et al., 2013). Simulation allows health professionals to practice clinical skills in a safe and controlled environment before they carry out the procedure or task on a real patient. It is important to distinguish simulators from simulation. Simulators can range from manikins that can mimic a complete patient, to part-task trainer simulators that simulate part of a body to allow a particular medical procedure to be practised (Levine et al., 2013). Simulation is a generic term that can include any activity that allows the learner to practice a skill or task outside of the real world. Simulation activities can include actors who play the role of a patient or real patients who are playing a role for the purpose of the learning session. Simulation can also include manikin-based simulators, or even computer-simulated patients.

It may be thought that the use of simulation in healthcare is a relatively recent phenomenon. However, simulators have been used in healthcare education and training for thousands of years. In fact, it has been suggested that the twentieth century was a 'dark age' for healthcare simulation as compared to the previous two centuries (Owen, 2012). For example, three hundred years ago France had a national simulation-based training curriculum for midwives in order to address Louis XV's worries about declining population numbers. An excellent overview of the widespread use of healthcare simulation up to the first years of the twentieth century is provided by Owen (2012).

In recent years, healthcare simulation technology has progressed rapidly, but so too has the educational and training techniques utilised. Such training has demonstrated positive outcomes and there is some evidence to support the transfer of learning to clinical practice with improved patient care and outcomes (Levine et al., 2013; McGaghie et al., 2011a). However, simulation can have impact beyond education and training and support a wide range of research and quality improvement applications.

PURPOSE OF THIS BOOK

The purpose of this book is to provide a foundational knowledge on how to:

1. design, deliver, and evaluate simulation-based education and training (Chapters 2–8);
2. run a simulation facility (Chapter 9); and
3. use simulation for research, and quality improvement (Chapters 10 and 11).

The content of this book is based upon the content of the Postgraduate Diploma and Masters in Healthcare Simulation and Patient Safety delivered at the University of Galway. This postgraduate educational programme was started by Professors O'Connor and Byrne in 2018. To date, we have had more than 300 graduates from a range of healthcare specialties (e.g., emergency medicine, surgery, anaesthesiology, obstetrics, psychiatry, general practice), with diverse roles (e.g., nurses, doctors, paramedics, simulation technicians, physiotherapists, medical physicists, veterinary practitioners), and from all over the world. This book draws upon the teaching materials, readings, and student feedback from this education programme and presents them in a single handbook that will be relevant for anyone interested in healthcare simulation.

CHAPTER OUTLINE

This opening chapter will:

- outline the ethical imperative of simulation-based education (SBE);
- describe the main categories of healthcare simulators;
- discuss simulation realism and why this is an important consideration in designing SBE;
- consider the evidence supporting the effectiveness of SBE; and
- provide an overview of some of the healthcare simulation societies, conferences, and journals.

ETHICAL IMPERATIVE OF SIMULATION-BASED EDUCATION

There is a fundamental tension in healthcare between the need for healthcare providers to practice their skills and the need for patients to be kept safe (Ziv et al., 2003). This tension can be alleviated through the use of simulation. Simulation offers the opportunity for healthcare providers to apply the knowledge they have learned through their formal education and practice the skills and techniques that are required to be a safe practitioner, in the context of a safe simulated environment. This environment will offer the opportunity to the healthcare provider to achieve an acceptable level of competence in a particular skill or procedure before they perform the task on a real patient. Simulation can never fully recreate the experience of delivering care to a real patient. Therefore, eventually all healthcare providers must develop their skills on real patients. However, there is an ethical and moral obligation upon the healthcare industry to ensure that healthcare providers have achieved a minimum level of competence before they 'practice' on a patient.

In other high-risk industries, simulation is commonly used to develop basic skills for novice learners. Training on a simulator provides an environment that allows a complete focus on the learner, without other distractions that may be present in the real environment. Moreover, simulation allows the learner to focus their attention on particular tasks or activities that they find difficult, and to repeat particular skills or procedural steps that they find challenging without having to complete the entire procedure. Using simulation to develop basic skills means that a learner can reach an acceptable level of proficiency before carrying out the task on a patient for the first time. Clearly, completing a clinical procedure in a simulated setting is not the same as performing the task on a real patient. However, the skills learned on the simulator has been shown to transfer to effective performance on a real patient. To illustrate, it has been shown that medical students require an average of five trials of venepuncture on a simulator (a total of 22 minutes of training) to learn how to perform all of the steps in the procedure correctly. Most importantly, these knowledge and skills transferred to a high-level performance on a real patient – all steps were performed with a minimum of 88% accuracy (Lydon et al., 2017).

Simulation also provides the opportunity for experienced healthcare providers to practice, and remain competent, in tasks or activities that they perform relatively rarely in the real world, but are very important (i.e., High Acuity Low Occurrence (HALO) events). This is a common way in which simulation is used in high-risk industries outside of healthcare. Applied to healthcare, regular practice, and feedback, in HALO events in a simulated setting can help to ensure that healthcare professionals are ready to effectively manage these events when they occur in the actual clinical environment. For example, it has been found that advance life support knowledge and skills decay six months to a year after training. Moreover, it has been found that advance life support skills decay faster than knowledge (Yang et al., 2012). Therefore, periodic simulation training can provide a mechanism to maintain competency in advanced life support skills.

Simulation can also be used to increase the efficiency of training. Increasing class sizes of undergraduate students, and a higher workload of clinical staff, means that students do not get the same opportunities to carry out clinical skills in the actual healthcare environment as may have been the case in the past. Moreover, even after graduation, training opportunities are more limited than was previously the case. Reasons for this change are shortening in the length of some graduate training programmes, and the implementation of working time limits such as the European Working Time Directive. SBE can address these limits of training time in the clinical environment. For example, it has been found that replacing half of traditional clinical placement hours with simulation had no significant impact on clinical competency, nursing knowledge, or licensing exam pass rate for US nursing students (Hayden et al., 2014).

TYPES OF HEALTHCARE SIMULATORS

There are a range of different types and modalities of healthcare simulators. We provide a brief description of the common types of healthcare simulators, and the advantages and disadvantages of each type, below. This list is not exhaustive, and terminology can differ. In this book we have largely adopted the nomenclature and definitions provided in the Healthcare Simulation Dictionary published by the Agency for Health Care Research and Quality and the Society for Simulation in Healthcare (Lioce et al., 2020).

MANIKIN SIMULATORS

These simulators are a 'plastic person' that uses computer algorithms to mimic the functions of a real patient. Manikin simulators can replicate: spontaneous breathing (and the ability to breathe for the patient with a bag or ventilator); real-time display of electronically monitored information (e.g., ECG, oxygen saturation); pulse, heart sounds, breath sounds, pupil size, pupil response to light; and obstruction to various parts of the airway. Generally speaking, the more money you spend, the greater the functionality of the simulator (but also the more potential for things to break). Manikin-based simulation allows learners to simultaneously practice a wide range of clinical and non-technical skills (e.g., decision-making, communication). For example, in the context of a particular patient presentation, learners can practice patient assessment, teamwork, decision-making, communication, seeking support, requesting investigations, reviewing results, and responding to deterioration.

- *Strengths*: supports the teaching of clinical and non-technical skills, can simulate a range of medical conditions.
- *Weaknesses*: requires an experienced team to run simulations, requires simulation technical operators, simulators can be expensive to purchase, bulky to store, learners may have difficulty engaging with the manikin as if it is a real patient, and very time-consuming to train large numbers of learners.

SIMULATED PARTICIPANTS

A Simulated Participant (SP) is a real person who has been trained to simulate a patient, relative, or healthcare provider. They can be patients (usually with a chronic condition) who are trained to support learning and assessment. In the past SPs were called standardised or simulated patients. SPs are distinct from a confederate, or embedded participant. An embedded participant is someone who plays a role in a simulation encounter to guide the scenario. The guidance may be positive or negative, or a distractor based on the objectives of the scenario (Lioce et al., 2020). The purpose of the embedded participant is to keep the scenario on track. They may wear an earpiece so they can receive direction from the control room. The change in the name recognises the broader role of SPs beyond assessment and playing patients. SPs can support practice, and assessment, of skills such as history taking, physical examination, and other clinical and non-technical skills. Generally, the main focus when engaging SPs is to practice or assess communication skills and to support learners to see things form the patients' perspectives.

- *Strengths*: high level of realism as the learner is interacting with a real person, effective approach to practice and assess communication skills.
- *Weaknesses*: SPs require extensive training, generally have to pay SPs, cannot easily simulate many medical conditions (e.g., arrhythmia).

TASK TRAINER/PART-TASK TRAINER

Task, or part-task, trainers are simulators designed to support the training of a particular clinical procedure (e.g., lumbar puncture, chest drain insertion; Levine et al., 2013). Task trainers generally consist of a model of a particular region or part of the body (e.g., arm, airway). They may be mechanical, electronic, or a combination of both. Therefore, the purpose of task trainers is to develop technical skills and to support teaching in how to perform a particular procedure.

- *Strengths*: can be used to develop technical skills and knowledge in a specific clinical procedure, large choice of different simulators in terms of capabilities and cost.
- *Weaknesses*: can be bulky to store, require maintenance and cleaning, generally can only simulate one procedure, and can only be used to teach technical skills.

Organic simulators. Organic simulators are derived from living matter such as animal tissue, or cadavers. Organic simulators are becoming less common as simulation technology improves. However, they are still important in particular specialities, such as surgery, where synthetic materials that provide realistic haptic feedback are lacking.

- *Strengths*: provide realistic haptic feedback, many animal specimens (e.g., pig bowel) are cheap and easily obtainable.
- *Weaknesses*: requires refrigerated storage facilities, messy, limits and regulations on the use of cadaveric specimens.

COMPUTER-BASED SIMULATORS

These simulators are run on a standard computer. These simulations can be described as in silico (Lioce et al., 2020). They use standard computer inputs (mouse, keyboard, and/or microphone) and outputs (a monitor) to carry out a range of simulations. For example, controlling an avatar in a virtual hospital setting, or interacting with a virtual patient. A particular type of computer-based simulation is a serious game. Serious games make use of a gaming approach to simulate real-world events, or processes designed for the purpose of solving a problem (see: www.breakawaygames.com for some examples). Although not generally relevant to SBE, computer simulations can also be used to support managerial and policy decisions (e.g., modelling the throughput of patients in an emergency department under different conditions, modelling the spread of a virus through a population).

- *Strengths*: computers are cheap and widely available, does not require special equipment, can be carried out at a place and time of the learners choosing, great flexibility in what is simulated, cost-effective approach for training large numbers of learners, performance and engagement can be monitored.
- *Weaknesses*: low realism and does not closely mimic a real clinical encounter, limited flexibility in the simulation, the teacher is unlikely to have input in how the simulation progresses as this is pre-programmed, learner receives limited feedback.

VIRTUAL REALITY SIMULATORS

Virtual reality is an advanced form of computer-based simulation that uses a wide range of immersive, and three-dimensional, visual cues to mimic real-life situations and/or healthcare procedures (Lioce et al., 2020). This type of simulation might involve wearing a special headset, or can be carried out in a room in which each surface is used as projection screens to create a highly immersive virtual environment called a CAVE (Cave Automatic Virtual Environment).

- *Strengths*: high level of realism, enthusiasm from learners to try the new technology.
- *Weaknesses*: expensive, largely a new technology so may still have some bugs, the teacher is unlikely to have input in how the simulation progresses as this is pre-programmed.

TABLE-TOP SIMULATION

This type of simulation is often used to simulate large-scale emergencies (e.g., plane crash). Personnel play particular emergency management roles in the simulation in order to test emergency plans and identify roles and responsibilities.

- *Strengths*: cheap, does not require a lot of technology.
- *Weaknesses*: low level of realism, only provides a relatively surface-level assessment of protocols.

One or more types of simulators described above can be used in one simulation event – this is known as *hybrid simulation*. The most common type of hybrid simulation is to combine SPs with a task trainer. For example, attaching an injection training pad to the arm of an SP. This combination provides the opportunity for the learner to practice both communicating with the patient, as well as performing a technical procedure. Another example of hybrid simulation is to incorporate an encounter with a relative in the context of a manikin-based simulation event.

Another distinction that is sometimes used to describe simulation is where it is carried out. Oftentimes, simulation is performed in an educational environment such as a simulation centre or facility separate from the clinical setting. However, if simulation is carried out in the actual setting where patient care is delivered (e.g., ICU, ambulance) then this is called *in situ simulation*. In situ simulation can be useful for assessing, troubleshooting, or developing new systems or processes (Lioce et al., 2020).

SIM ZONES

Instead of considering simulations in terms of type of simulator used, as delineated above, it might instead be useful to categorise them based upon learning needs. Sim Zones is a system for organising simulations and matching different types of simulation activities to particular learning needs (Roussin & Weinstock, 2017). This approach divides simulation activities into five distinct zones which describe the purpose of the simulation, the resources and staff skill set and the approach to learner feedback:

- *Zone 0: Auto-feedback* responds to the need for learners to practice procedural skills. As the name suggests, feedback is automatic and is based on performance on the virtual reality simulator which can be done remotely, by solitary learners, and without an instructor present.
- *Zone 1: Foundational instruction* is the next level up in terms of activity, learner groups and feedback. In this zone, the goals are learning and practicing how, and occasionally what and when, to do something according to standard practice. The learner usually has the opportunity to practice the skill (ideally with the opportunity for repeated practice), under the observation of the instructor and receive individualised feedback on performance to guide development. Zone 1 simulations can be embedded into larger training programmes (e.g., clinical orientations) and may involve rotating stations.
- *Zone 2: Acute situational instruction* is a type of simulation event that is designed to promote learning of contextualised clinical skills (e.g., identifying a deteriorating patient and escalating care). Sometimes these simulation events involve partial or full clinical teams, but may also involve any group of learners that would benefit from practicing acute clinical events. Typically zone 2 simulations involve an embedded participant who will role play with a manikin and/or simulated participants.
- *Zone 3: Team and systems development* simulations are carried out with real designated clinical teams with a focus on team and system development. Often these simulations are concerned with the management of high-risk scenarios by a multi-disciplinary team (e.g., massive blood transfusion). The focus of these simulations is generally on improving the response to these scenarios by considering the range of factors that contribute to good, or poor, performance. This may cover the performance of the team itself, but also issues with procedures and protocols, equipment, or the environment. Such simulations may be carried out in a designated simulation centre, but they may also be carried out in situ (i.e., the simulation takes place in the actual patient care setting/environment).
- *Zone 4: Real-life debriefing and development* is focused on debriefing after a real patient event – using the same approach as in zone 3. This zone is not really simulation, but these real events can be used to create zone 3 simulations.

SIMULATION AND REALISM

Within the context of healthcare simulation, realism has been defined as: "the ability to impart the suspension of disbelief to the learner by creating an environment that mimics that of the learner's work environment; realism includes the environment, simulated patient, and activities of the educators, assessors, and/or facilitators" (Lioce et al., 2020: 41). A term that is often used synonymously with realism is fidelity – although it is not universally agreed that these two concepts are the same.

Fidelity can be defined as the extent to which the simulation event replicates the actual clinical environment (Alessi, 1988). Simulators tend to be described as either low or high fidelity depending on how closely they represent the real world. High fidelity refers to simulation experiences that are very realistic and provide a level of interactivity and realism for the learner that is very close to what is experienced in the real clinical environment (Lioce et al., 2020). From a teaching perspective, three broad dimensions of fidelity should be considered.

- *Equipment fidelity*. The degree to which the simulation duplicates the equipment that is actually used in the clinical environment.
- *Environmental fidelity*. The extent to which the simulation duplicates the visual, auditory, and haptic (i.e., touch and feel) cues in the clinical environment.
- *Psychological fidelity*. The extent to which the simulation mimics the psychological and cognitive factors that are present in the real clinical environment such that the learner can suspend disbelief and react in the simulation as they would in the real clinical environment.

The extent to which each domain of fidelity is important is dependent upon the type of simulation that is being carried out. To illustrate, psychological fidelity is particularly important for team training. If the learners do not suspend their disbelief, then they are unlikely to behave in the simulation as they would in the real world (Beaubien & Baker, 2004). In contrast, when learning basic clinical skills, equipment and environmental fidelity are more important. The learner should use the same equipment that is used to carry out the procedure, and get the same haptic feedback as they would feel if performing the procedure on a patient. However, it is important to make the point that there is not necessarily a strong correlation between fidelity and learning outcomes.

It has been found that training outcomes using high-fidelity simulation are comparable to those achieved using lower-fidelity simulation. Any differences in favour of high-fidelity simulation are modest and tend not to be statistically significant (Lefor et al., 2020; Norman et al., 2012; Sherwood & Francis, 2018). The Alessi hypothesis states that there is a point at which increasing fidelity does not have an impact on training outcomes, and may even have a negative impact on learning outcomes (Alessi, 1988). Alessi (1988) proposes that the lack of a large effect of increased fidelity is due to:

(1) high-fidelity simulation increases the complexity of the simulation for the learner (e.g., more distractions, higher workload), and so impedes learning; and
(2) high-fidelity simulation being 'wasted' on inexperienced learners who can learn through effective instruction on less distracting low-fidelity simulations.

Therefore, both learner experience, and the dimensions of fidelity, are important considerations when designing simulation-based education.

Hamstra et al. (2014) propose that the term fidelity should be abandoned, and that there is a need for a greater focus on what is defined as functional task alignment. This is particularly true when describing a simulator as 'low' or 'high' fidelity, since these terms do not have clear definitions (Cook et al., 2011). Moreover, to add further confusion, there are contextual issues which may mean some aspects of a simulator could be considered high fidelity, and others low fidelity. Therefore, Hamstra et al. (2014) recommend that rather than focusing on fidelity, simulationists should instead consider the functional task alignment of the simulator. So, rather than a focus on what the simulator looks like, it should be considered in terms of the functional properties of the simulator and how these align with the learning objectives of a particular SBE activity. Regardless of whether or not you wish to use the term fidelity, this alignment is a crucial consideration when deciding on the most appropriate simulator to use.

EFFECTIVENESS OF SIMULATION

Although there is more acceptance of the use of healthcare simulation than there was even a decade ago, a 'burden of proof' that healthcare simulation is effective seems to persist. This has led to authors identifying a need for high-quality studies, such as randomised controlled trials, in order to identify the impact of simulation on patient outcomes (e.g., Meling & Meling, 2021; So et al., 2019). Smith and Pell (2003) published a clever 'tongue-in-cheek' article entitled 'parachute use to prevent death and major trauma due to gravitational challenge'. The authors used the absence of any randomised controlled trials in testing the effectiveness of parachutes to prevent major trauma, to make the point that situations exist where trials may not be required and/or appropriate. It is certainly true that there have been a limited number of randomised controlled trials of the impact of simulation on clinical outcomes. However, even if there is limited evidence for the impact of simulation on clinical outcomes, there is a large volume of data supporting the positive impact of simulation on the knowledge, skills, and behaviour of learners (Cook et al., 2011; McGaghie et al., 2011b; McGaghie et al., 2010; Walsh et al., 2018). It is also noteworthy that there is considerably more evidence to support the use of simulation in healthcare as compared to aviation. This is despite the fact that simulation has been commonplace in aviation for almost a century.

Even if funding were to be available to conduct trials on the effect of simulation, the questions is not as simple as 'Does healthcare simulation work?' The current questions on simulation effectiveness are open-ended and much more nuanced (Walsh et al., 2018). These include questions like 'Why, how, and with whom does healthcare simulation work?'; 'How much simulation is required to make an impact?'; and 'What is the cost-effectiveness of different types of simulation-based education programmes?'. It is important to consider that it is almost impossible to isolate the impact of SBE from the huge number of other factors that impact clinical outcomes. Therefore, there is no simple direct link between SBE and clinical outcomes. The effects of SBE are modulated by a huge range of factors such as the culture of the organisation, buy-in from staff, the education skills of the teachers, the appropriateness of the outcome measure, and so on. Therefore, we strongly caution against using patient outcomes as the only measure of the impact of a SBE programme. The evaluation of simulation-based education is discussed in much more detail in Chapter 3, and using simulation for research in Chapter 10.

HEALTHCARE SIMULATION SOCIETIES AND CONFERENCES

There is a growing community of people interested in healthcare simulation supported by many societies and conferences. Healthcare simulation societies provide opportunities to learn, share, and network with others with an interest in simulation. It is also possible to become accredited as an individual, or centre, by many of these societies. Most societies hold an annual conference, as well as other networking and education events. These conferences are a useful forum to network with other simulationists, attend workshops on simulation, and hear about/present simulation research or Quality Improvement projects. The conferences also have large exhibitions in which the simulation equipment manufacturers show their latest simulators.

There are many different simulation societies. These include societies focused on a particular professional group (e.g., *International Nursing Association for Clinical Simulation and Learning*; *Society of Surgical Simulation*), or country (e.g., *Irish Association for Simulation*, *Australian Society for Simulation in Healthcare*). These societies are too numerous to discuss here. However, below is a list of some of the bigger interprofessional simulation societies.

- *Society for Simulation in Healthcare (SSH)*: www.ssih.org. SSH is a US-based simulation society that was founded in 2004. The goal of SSH is to promote improvements in simulation technology, educational methods, practitioner assessment, and patient safety that promote better patient care and can improve patient outcome. The SSH annual conference is held at the beginning of each year in one of the major US conference venues.
- *Association for Simulated Practice in Healthcare (ASPiH)*: aspih.org.uk. ASPiH is a UK-based simulation society. The goals of ASPiH are to: provide a communication network for those involved in simulation; provide examples of best practice in education, training, assessment and research in healthcare; support the expansion and uptake of

simulation; develop and share key operational and strategic resources; encourage and support the dissemination of innovative practice in simulation; and become the 'go-to' independent organisation for those looking for information about healthcare simulation. The ASPiH annual conference is held towards the end of the year in rotating UK cities.

- *Society in Europe for Simulation Applied to Medicine (SESAM)*: www.sesam-web.org The mission of SESAM is to encourage and support the use of simulation in healthcare for the purpose of training and research. The SESAM annual conference is held in different cities in Europe during the summer.

HEALTHCARE SIMULATION JOURNALS

There are a number of peer-reviewed healthcare simulation journals that publish a range of research, reviews, and guidance on healthcare simulation. These journals include:

- *Simulation in Healthcare*: journals.lww.com/simulationinhealthcare/. This is the journal of the SSH. It is a multi-disciplinary publication that covers all areas of applications and research in healthcare simulation technology.
- *Advances in Simulation*: advancesinsimulation.biomedcentral.com/. This is the journal of SESAM. The aim of this journal is to provide a forum to share scholarly practice to advance the use of simulation in health and social care. This journal is open-access. This means that the articles are freely available for anyone to access. However, this means that there is generally a fee to publish in the journal (although this can be waived in certain situations).
- *International Journal of Healthcare Simulation* – Advances in Theory and Practice: www. ijohs.com/. This open-access journal also provides a forum to share scholarly practice for advances in simulation across health and social care.
- *Clinical Simulation in Nursing*: www.nursingsimulation.org. This is the journal of the International Nursing Association for Clinical Simulation and Learning. The aim of the journal is to advance the science of healthcare simulation.
- *Journal of Surgical Simulation*: www.journalsurgicalsimulation.com/. This is the journal of the Society for Surgical Simulation. The journal is focused on publishing research in the field of surgical simulation and surgical education.

Healthcare education journals, such as *Medical Teacher*, *Medical Education* and the *Journal of Nursing Education*, also publish simulation research. Simulation papers may also be published in specialty-specific journals.

CONCLUSION

Healthcare simulation is the modern way to educate healthcare providers to achieve high performance and to improve patient safety and quality of care. It is an experiential approach to teaching the technical and non-technical skills required by healthcare professionals. However, the simulators themselves are only educational tools. As discussed in the subsequent chapters of this book, although important, the simulators are only one part of designing an effective healthcare simulation programme.

FURTHER READING

Hamstra, S. J., Brydges, R., Hatala, R., Zendejas, B., Cook, D. A. (2014). Reconsidering fidelity in simulation-based training. *Academic Medicine*, 89(3), 387–392.

Lioce, L. (Ed.). et al. (2020). *Healthcare Simulation Dictionary*. Rockville, MD: Agency for Healthcare Research and Quality. Available from: https://www.ssih.org/Dictionary.

Owen, H. (2012). Early use of simulation in medical education. *Simulation in Healthcare*, 7(2), 102–116.

Roussin, C. J., Weinstock, P. (2017). SimZones: an organizational innovation for simulation programs and centers. *Academic Medicine*, *92*, 1114–1120.

Ziv, A., Wolpe, P. R., Small, S. D., Glick, S. (2003). Simulation-based medical education: an ethical imperative. *Academic Medicine*, *78*(8), 783–788.

ONLINE RESOURCES

- Healthy simulation: www.healthysimulation.com large range of resources on healthcare simulation.
- SimGHOST is an organisation with resources on simulation with a simulation technician focus: simghosts.org.
- Examples of healthcare simulation manufacturing companies include:
  - CAE healthcare: www.caehealthcare.com.
  - Gaumard: www.gaumard.com.
  - Laerdal: laerdal.com.
  - Limbs and Things: limbsandthings.com/global.
  - Simulab: simulab.com/.

REFERENCES

Alessi, S. M. (1988). Fidelity in the design of instructional simulations. *Journal of Computer-Based Instruction*, *15*(2), 40–47.

Beaubien, J. M., Baker, D. P. (2004). The use of simulation for training teamwork skills in health care: how low can you go? *BMJ Quality & Safety*, *13*(suppl 1), i51–i56.

Cook, D. A., Hatala, R., Brydges, R., Zendejas, B., Szostek, J. H., Wang, A. T., … Hamstra, S. J. (2011). Technology-enhanced simulation for health professions education: a systematic review and meta-analysis. *Journal of the American Medical Association*, *306*(9), 978–988.

Hamstra, S. J., Brydges, R., Hatala, R., Zendejas, B., Cook, D. A. (2014). Reconsidering fidelity in simulation-based training. *Academic Medicine*, *89*(3), 387–392.

Hayden, J. K., Smiley, R. A., Alexander, M., Kardong-Edgren, S., Jeffries, P. R. (2014). The NCSBN national simulation study: a longitudinal, randomized, controlled study replacing clinical hours with simulation in prelicensure nursing education. *Journal of Nursing Regulation*, *5*(2), S3–S40.

Lefor, A. K., Harada, K., Kawahira, H., Mitsuishi, M. (2020). The effect of simulator fidelity on procedure skill training: a literature review. *International Journal of Medical Education*, *11*, 97–106.

Levine, A. I., DeMaria Jr, S., Schwartz, A. D., Sim, A. J. (Eds.) (2013). *The Comprehensive Textbook of Healthcare Simulation*. Berlin, Germany: Springer Science & Business Media.

Lioce, L. J. L., Downing, D., Chang, T. P., Robertson, J. M., Anderson, M., … the Terminology and Concepts Working Group (Eds.). (2020). *Healthcare Simulation Dictionary - Second Edition*. Rockville, MD: Agency for Healthcare Research and Quality.

Lydon, S., Burns, N., Healy, O., O'Connor, P., McDermott, B. R., Byrne, D. (2017). Preliminary evaluation of the efficacy of an intervention incorporating precision teaching to train procedural skills among final cycle medical students. *BMJ Simulation & Technology Enhanced Learning*, *3*(3), 116.

McGaghie, W. C., Draycott, T. J., Dunn, W. F., Lopez, C. M., Stefanidis, D. (2011a). Evaluating the impact of simulation on translational patient outcomes. *Simulation in Healthcare*, *6*(Suppl), S42–S7.

McGaghie, W. C., Issenberg, S. B., Cohen, E. R., Barsuk, J. H., Wayne, B. (2011b). Does simulation-based medical education with deliberate practice yield better results than traditional clinical education? A meta-analytic comparative review of the evidence. *Academic Medicine*, *86*(6), 706–711.

McGaghie, W. C., Issenberg, S. B., Petrusa, E. R., & Scalese, R. J. (2010). A critical review of simulation-based medical education research: 2003-2009. *Medical Education*, *44*(1), 50–63.

Meling, T. R., Meling, T. R. (2021). The impact of surgical simulation on patient outcomes: a systematic review and meta-analysis. *Neurosurgical Review*, *44*(2), 843–854.

Norman, G., Dore, K., Grierson, L. (2012). The minimal relationship between simulation fidelity and transfer of learning. *Medical Education*, *46*(7), 636–647.

Owen, H. (2012). Early use of simulation in medical education. *Simulation in Healthcare*, 7(2), 102–116.

Roussin, C. J., Weinstock, P. (2017). SimZones: an organizational innovation for simulation programs and centers. *Academic Medicine*, *92*(8), 1114–1120.

Sherwood, R. J., Francis, G. (2018). The effect of mannequin fidelity on the achievement of learning outcomes for nursing, midwifery and allied healthcare practitioners: Systematic review and meta-analysis. *Nurse Education Today*, *69*, 81–94.

Smith, G. C., Pell, J. P. (2003). Parachute use to prevent death and major trauma related to gravitational challenge: systematic review of randomised controlled trials. *British Medical Journal*, *327*(7429), 1459–1461.

So, H. Y., Chen, P. P., Wong, G. K. C., Chan, T. T. N. (2019). Simulation in medical education. *Journal of the Royal College of Physicians of Edinburgh*, *49*(1), 52–57.

Walsh, C., Lydon, S., Byrne, D., Madden, C., Fox, S., O'Connor, P. (2018). The 100 most cited articles on healthcare simulation: a bibliometric review. *Simulation in Healthcare*, *13*(3), 211–220.

Yang, C.-W., Yen, Z.-S., McGowan, J. E., Chen, H. C., Chiang, W.-C., Mancini, M. E., … Ma, M. H.-M. (2012). A systematic review of retention of adult advanced life support knowledge and skills in healthcare providers. *Resuscitation*, *83*(9), 1055–1060.

Ziv, A., Wolpe, P. R., Small, S. D., Glick, S. (2003). Simulation-based medical education: an ethical imperative. *Academic Medicine*, *78*(8), 783–788.

2 Learning Theories

INTRODUCTION

A theory seeks to explain why, or how, something occurs. The purpose of a learning theory is to generate an understanding of how knowledge is created, a skill is acquired, and how people gained this knowledge or skill. Many educators begin teaching with little knowledge of learning theory. They apply the educational approaches they experienced as learners, or methods that their learners seem to like. Therefore, while it is possible to teach with little knowledge of learning theory, there are benefits to having (at least some) understanding of learning theories and what they can offer the educator in designing and delivering education and training. It is fair to say that learning theory is often not being applied to the design of simulation-based education (SBE). In a review of the application of theory-based research to the use of high-fidelity simulation in nursing education it was found that almost half of the studies reviewed made no use of theory, and only 10% of the studies were categorised as 'adequately theory-based' (Rourke et al., 2010).

Artino and Konopasky (2018) provide two practical reasons as to why learning theory is useful to educators. Firstly, learning theory provides a framework to support the design of instruction. Learning theory can provide explanations as to why, and under what circumstances, particular teaching methods are effective or ineffective. Secondly, learning theory can help educators design instruction that is founded upon empirically tested principles – rather than based upon the learning experiences of the teacher.

CHAPTER OUTLINE

There is no single unified education theory that can be applied to all of SBE. It is also beyond the scope of this chapter to review every educational theory that could be relevant to SBE. Therefore, this chapter will discuss four different learning theories that are commonly discussed within the context of SBE. These theories are: (1) adult learning theory; (2) behavioural learning theory; (3) social cognitive learning theory; and (4) constructivist learning theory. Finally, an approach to SBE – called mastery training – will be discussed that draws upon all of these learning theories.

DOI: 10.1201/9781003296942-2

ADULT LEARNING THEORY

The participants in SBE are generally adult learners. In the 1960s Malcolm Knowles proposed a theory of adult learning called andragogy – which continues to influence education and learning today. Andragogy is concerned with the art and science of helping adults to learn. Knowles identified five assumptions about adult learning:

1. adults are independent and self-directing;
2. adult learners have accumulated a great deal of experience which they bring to the educational setting;
3. adult learners value learning that integrates with the demands of their everyday lives;
4. adult learners are more interested in immediate, problem-centred approaches than in subject-centred ones; and
5. adult learners are more motivated to learn by internal drives than by external ones.

(Kaufman, 2003)

Knowles then built upon these assumptions and proposed seven principles of andragogy. These seven principles are:

1. establish an effective learning climate, where learners feel safe and comfortable expressing themselves;
2. involve learners in diagnosing their own needs – this will help to trigger internal motivation;
3. encourage learners to formulate their own learning objectives – this gives them more control of their learning;
4. involve learners in mutual planning of relevant methods and curricular content;
5. encourage learners to identify resources and devise strategies for using the resources to achieve their objectives;
6. support learners in carrying out their learning plans; and
7. involve learners in evaluating their own learning – this can develop their skills of critical reflection.

(Kaufman, 2003)

It has been argued that andragogy is not really a theory at all, but a philosophy based on self-directed, independent learning methods for adults. This philosophy underpins many adult learning theories – including those described in this chapter.

BEHAVIOURAL LEARNING THEORY

Behavioural learning theory proposes that all behaviours are learned through interaction with the environment. This learning theory is founded upon the experiments conducted by the Russian psychologist Ivan Pavlov in the 1890s. Pavlov demonstrated that he was able to condition dogs to salivate at the sound of a bell. He achieved this effect by ringing a bell when the dogs were given food. After a number of repeated trials, he found that ringing the bell (stimulus) resulted in the dog salivating (response) when there was no food. Behaviourism is founded upon three assumptions:

1. the behaviour to be learned is observable;
2. the environment shapes the behaviour; and
3. reinforcement (e.g., through feedback) is fundamental to the learning process.

(Torre et al., 2006)

When constructing SBE using a behaviourist approach, it is necessary to identify exactly what behaviour(s) the learner is expected to *perform*, the *conditions* under which the learner is expected to perform the behaviour(s), and the criteria for acceptable performance of the behaviour. For example, a final year medical student will carry out venepuncture (performance) in a simulated setting (condition), with 100% accuracy within a maximum time of 10 minutes (criteria). As compared to the learning theories discussed below, behaviourist approaches are a teacher-centric approach to learning. The teacher controls the learning environment in order to support the learner to achieve the desired response (Torre et al., 2006). Given the focus on very well-defined and observable behaviour, behaviourist approaches are particularly applicable to teaching clinical procedural skills using strategies such as deliberate practice or precision teaching – described below.

DELIBERATE PRACTICE

In the early 1990s, Ericsson et al. (1993) published a study identifying the most effective form of musical instrument training. This study found that the most effective form of training used individualised lessons for each learner, with associated goals to guide the learner's own practice between lessons. Based on the findings of this paper, Malcolm Gladwell proposed that approximately 10,000 hours of practice are required to be an expert in any given task (Gladwell, 2008). Ericsson estimated that, in fact, winning an international piano competition requires approximately 25,000 hours of practice (Ericsson, 2013). However, regardless of the exact number of hours of practice necessary, the key requirements of deliberate practice are sustained hours of practice, hard work, feedback, and perseverance under exacting conditions (McGaghie et al., 2021). It is clear that many of the strategies that are currently relied upon for training healthcare professionals do not meet the criteria for deliberate practice. For example, observing a procedure being performed is not deliberate practice. In order to learn effectively, the learner must actually conduct the procedure with direct feedback from a supervisor. Ideally, then practicing the procedure in a simulated setting before the next supervised teaching session.

McGaghie et al. (2020) identified a bundle of ten integrated components of deliberate practice. These components are:

1. the learner is very motivated to master the task/procedure;
2. the task/procedure to be taught is clear, with well-defined learning objectives;
3. the level of difficulty is appropriate for the proposed learners;
4. practice is both focused and deliberate;
5. there are rigorous, precise, and reliable measurements of performance of the task/procedure;
6. feedback on performance is provided to the learner by a teacher;
7. learners monitor their own learning (e.g., identify and address errors) and then engage in more deliberate practice;
8. learners are assessed to ensure they have met the desired standard;
9. the learner continues on to master a different task/procedure; and
10. the learner has a goal of constant improvement.

(McGaghie et al., 2020)

Unsurprisingly, many studies exploring the efficacy of deliberate practice as a learning strategy have made use of simulation. A simulated setting is the ideal environment for such research as it provides a safe and controlled environment for learners to practice, undergo rigorous assessment of their performance, and receive feedback. There is a large body of research on the effectiveness of deliberate practice (see McGaghie et al., 2011a).

More recently, deliberate practice has been adapted into what has been defined as rapid cycle deliberate practice (see Example 2.1). In rapid cycle deliberate practice, a simulated task/experience is divided into less complex parts and each individual part is repeatedly practiced with rapid debriefing cycles until expert performance is obtained (Rosman et al., 2019). The simulated task/experience then moves onto the next step or level of difficulty. In rapid cycle deliberate practice:

- there are "real-time" interruptions in the simulation to facilitate immediate corrections of "bad habits/errors" to support the development of new skills through repetition and practice;
- a safe learning environment is established in order to support the learner to address doubts by asking questions; and
- new information is divided into small chunks to prevent the learner becoming overloaded and to reinforce learning in real time.

(Chancey et al., 2019)

EXAMPLE 2.1   THE USE OF RAPID CYCLE DELIBERATE PRACTICE TO TEACH DEATH NOTIFICATION

A rapid cycle deliberate practice technique of micro-debriefing (pause, debrief, rewind and try again) was used to teach 22 Emergency Medicine residents to deliver a death notification to a simulated participant playing the role of a relative of the deceased (Ahmed et al., 2020). After a period of didactic teaching on the subject, the learners carried out a complete, and uninterrupted, delivery of a death notification to a simulated participant. This simulated experience was followed by a high-level micro-debrief of the learners' performance. The learner then repeated the same simulated experience. However, this time the teacher paused the scenario to provide feedback (either to reinforce positive performance or provide constructive feedback), or to 'rewind' the scenario, and then restart the simulation. Intermittently the teacher also 'tagged in' another observing learner by switching out the learner in the simulation during a pause. The scenario was then repeated for a third and final time, using the same pause, debrief, rewind and try again approach. It was found that there was a significant improvement in performance and self-efficacy of the 22 learners who participated in the study (Ahmed et al., 2020).

PRECISION TEACHING

Another example of a behaviourist approach to learning is precision teaching (see Example 2.2). Precision teaching was first applied in special education teaching sessions with children. However, this teaching approach has now been applied in a wide range of settings, including medical education.

EXAMPLE 2.2   APPLICATION OF PRECISION TEACHING

In this study SBE and precision teaching were used to teach venepuncture to medical students (Lydon et al., 2017). The intervention consisted of timed learning trials during which participants carried out the skill in pairs and received corrective feedback. Intervention group participants required an average of five trials and 21.9 minutes to reach the fluency criterion of completing the procedure with 100% accuracy in 4.5 minutes. The time was based upon the time taken for an experienced phlebotomist to complete the task (+10%).

The intervention group demonstrated significantly higher accuracy in venepuncture performance than the control groups that did not receive the training. These improvements remained eight weeks after the training, did not deteriorate during distraction (answering questions while doing the task), and generalised to improved performance with real patients and peripheral intravenous cannulation (Lydon et al., 2017).

There are many similarities between deliberate practice and precision teaching. Both approaches are founded upon clear objectives, repeated practice, feedback, and performance assessment. However, the goal of precision teaching is to build behavioural fluency. Behavioural fluency can be defined as the "combination of accuracy plus speed of responding that enables competent individuals to function efficiently and effectively in their natural environment" (Binder, 1996). This focus on fluency extends the notion of accuracy of task performance by adding consideration of pacing or flow.

On completion of the training, the learner is expected to accurately perform the steps of the procedure within a timeframe close to that of an expert. Individuals that have learned a behaviour to fluency can: Retain the ability to perform the behaviour for long periods of time; Endure performing the skill for longer durations; Adapt the behaviour to part of a new, more complex, compound behaviour; Perform the skill at a rate that makes it functional; and maintain the performance of the skill even when distracted – described as Stability (REAPS; Kubina & Yurich, 2012). There is little to be gained in performing a procedure correctly if it takes an extremely long time to do so. Precision teaching aims to build automaticity in performance such that a task can be performed rapidly, without the need for great concentration. As such, once fluency has been attained it should be possible to complete the task with little conscious effort – even when the training was completed a long time ago.

TASK ANALYSIS

It can be seen that behavioural learning approaches require the establishment of a standard for task performance. This can be achieved through the use of human reliability analysis (HRA) techniques (Kirwan & Ainsworth, 1992). HRA consists of approaches to standardise task performance, systematically identify the impact of human error on a system, and to identify 'a correct way' for completing a procedure. Task analysis is a particular HRA technique that has been identified as an appropriate method of identifying the steps required to complete a procedure. There are many types of task analysis (see Kirwan & Ainsworth, 1992). However, the purpose of them all is to deconstruct procedures into a series of smaller steps (or sub-goals) that must be followed in order to complete the procedure (Lavelle et al., 2020). A commonly used three-stage approach to conducting a task analysis is:

1. conduct a literature search in order to identify if there is an existing task analysis of the procedure of interest that could be used or adapted;
2. conduct direct observation of subject matter experts (SMEs) performing the procedure in the real, or simulated, clinical environment; and
3. show the draft task analysis derived from stages 1 and 2 to a small group of SMEs in order to reach a consensus on 'a correct way' for completing the procedure.

(Reddy et al., 2020)

An excerpt from a task analysis of the nasogastric tube insertion procedure is shown in Example 2.3. Another important consideration to address in stage 3 of the task analysis is the level of detail that is required. By way of illustration, the detail of how to perform hand hygiene is not described in Example 2.3.

SOCIAL COGNITIVE LEARNING THEORY

Social cognitive learning theory is based upon the premise that learning is a social process that occurs in a social context. This theory is derived from the research carried out by Albert Bandura on the aggressive behaviour of children. A particularly well-known experiment carried out by Bandura and colleagues is called the Bobo doll experiment (Bandura, 1977). In this experiment, a group of preschool children watched a video in which an adult aggressively attacked a plastic inflated

EXAMPLE 2.3   PREPARATION OF PATIENT STEPS FOR NASOGASTRIC TUBE INSERTION*

4. Perform hand hygiene	• Perform the eight steps of hand hygiene as outlined by the World Health Organization.
5. Position the patient	• Ask the patient to sit in an upright position and to slightly flex their neck. Ask for assistance if required.
6. Measure the ngt	• Measure the NGT by placing the tip of the tube at the nostril, bringing the length towards the patient's ear and then to the xiphisternum. • Add 10cm to this measurement. • Note the measured length – you may mark this with a piece of tape.
7. Check patient's nostril patency	• Ask the patient to occlude one nostril with their finger and then to sniff in to demonstrate patency of that nostril. Then ask them to repeat with the other nostril. • If there is any evidence of obstruction, select the nostril that appears most patent. If both appear to be of limited patency, seek senior advice before proceeding.
8. Arrange a signal to allow the patient to communicate with you during the procedure	• Inform the patient that they should not speak/try to speak during the procedure and that you will require them to swallow as best they can when you are inserting the tube. • You may decide in collaboration with the patient, what signal they will use to indicate that they are distressed, for example, the patient raising their hand. However, note that if a NGT enters the lung, a patient in distress may not be able to communicate in this manner and the healthcare professional performing the procedure should be mindful of the patient's body language throughout the insertion.

* see Reid-McDermott et al. (2022) for a complete outline of the steps for this procedure.

clown called the Bobo doll. The children who watched this aggressive behaviour were also found to behave violently towards the Bobo doll, whereas children who were not exposed to the video of the adult behaving aggressively to the doll did not. This led to Bandura concluding that new behaviours could be learned in the absence of reward, or practice but through a combination of internal forces – cognition, and social forces such as observation, imitation and modelling (Bandura, 1977). Social cognitive learning theory builds upon the earlier behaviourist learning theory but crucially, adds the following premise – mediating processes take place between stimulus and response (i.e., human cognition) and behaviour can be learned through observation of the environment. Thus, the theory proposes that cognition, behaviour, and the environment are inter-linked and impact learning (Bandura, 1977).

Cognition is very important in the theory and Bandura proposed the concept of human agency as being central to learning (Bandura, 1986). Human agency is a person's capacity to determine how they respond to a particular situation. This determination is based upon self-efficacy and self-regulation. Both of these concepts are key to social cognitive learning theory (Bandura, 1986). Self-efficacy is the learner's belief that they have the knowledge and ability to manage a particular situation. From a SBE perspective, this means that complexity or difficulty of a scenario should be aligned to a learner's ability. The purpose of the SBE is to build the learner's confidence to manage the same, or a similar, situation in the actual clinical environment. Therefore, in SBE that is based upon social cognitive learning theory, self-efficacy is a product of the educational programme (McGaghie & Harris, 2018).

Self-regulation is concerned with the learner's ability to regulate their own learning and behaviour, set goals for achievement, and direct their behaviour accordingly. SBE builds on the principle of self-regulation by supporting and encouraging learners to set personal goals and strategies for the achievement of those goals. Learners are supported with planning, practicing, monitoring and reflecting on performance within the SBE environment.

CONSTRUCTIVIST LEARNING THEORY

Constructivist learning theory asserts that learners construct knowledge rather than passively taking in information. Learning is recognised to be a naturally occurring activity, with individuals constructing knowledge and meaning based upon their own perceptions, interpretations, conceptual constructs, existing knowledge and experience. New knowledge is incorporated into pre-existing knowledge schemas (McGaghie & Harris, 2018). Constructivist educational approaches are 'learner-centred'. The goal of the teacher is not to directly instruct the learner; rather, the teacher facilitates the self-directed learning and reflections of the learner. A particular influential constructivist perspective that is very pertinent to SBE is experiential learning.

EXPERIENTIAL LEARNING

Experiential learning theory is holistic learning theory in which experience plays a central role. According to Kolb's experiential learning theory (Kolb, 1984), knowledge is created through experience. Reflection is used to assimilate the experience and create new knowledge. Abstract conceptualisation involves integrating new learning into existing knowledge structures and active experimentation involves using these new knowledge structures to make decisions and solve problems. This process will lead to further concrete experience in a positive cycle of learning.

Experience plays a central role in experiential learning theory. Experiential learning proposes that learning is derived from meaning developed from direct experience. Experiential learning has its roots in the work of Kolb (1984) and others who espouse 'learning by doing' as a powerful approach to education. Given that healthcare simulation is focused upon the same premise, experiential learning fits well with SBE. One of the most influential models of experiential learning is Kolb's experiential learning cycle (see Figure 2.1). In the model, Kolb proposes that learning is

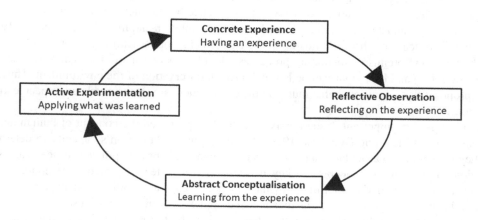

FIGURE 2.1   Kolb's experiential learning cycle.

cyclical – "thoughts are formed and re-formed through experience... learning is a process whereby concepts are derived from and continuously modified by experience" (Kolb, 1984: 26).

- *Concrete experience.* A real, or simulated, experience is the beginning of the learning process. In SBE, essential aspects of the clinical environment are replicated using tools and techniques such as manikin simulators, standardised patients or task trainers. The requirement for the learner to engage and perform the simulated task or activity provides the concrete experience. Ideally, this will be as an active participant rather than as an observer. Experience itself is important but it is the reflection on and application of the experience in the later phases where the powerful learning occurs.
- *Reflective observation.* Reflective observation can occur during and/or after the simulated experience. Often it occurs during the debriefing following the simulation when the debriefer encourages the learner to reflect on their performance and on the drivers of performance (see Chapter 7 for a discussion of debriefing). The learner reflects on what occurred during the simulated experience. The goal of the reflection is to encourage the learner to consider the drivers of their performance and to uncover the frames or mental models that may underlie the actions or decisions that they took. A skilled debriefer can help to uncover flawed or faulty frames that lead to inappropriate actions. Uncovering these faulty frames will lead the learner to change how they approach the same (or a similar) situation in the future (Zigmont et al., 2011).
- *Abstract conceptualisation.* In this stage the learner builds on the experience and reflection that occurred in the previous stages, and integrates the learning that has occurred into existing knowledge structures. Furthermore, the learner considers the implications of learning that has occurred on future experiences or to different contexts or situations (Zigmont et al., 2011). This stage can be facilitated by the debriefer by asking the learner how the simulated experience will impact their decisions or actions in the clinical environment.
- *Active experimentation.* In this stage, the learner applies what has been learned to make decisions or take action, either in the actual clinical environment or in the simulation environment. Evidence suggests that, if possible, learners should be allowed the opportunity to immediately apply their learning in the simulated environment. Immediate active experimenting supports the "cementing" of new knowledge/ways of working and supports long-term changes in clinical practice (Zigmont et al., 2011).

All four elements of experiential learning should be included in the phases of the simulation design and, furthermore, that active participation in all phases of the simulation experience is essential, so the learner becomes aware of each phase of the learning processes. Evidence suggests that the simulation experience itself and reflective debriefing are generally well implemented in simulation. However, the elements of abstract conceptualisation (thinking) and active experimentation (planning) are often omitted from simulation experiences in healthcare, or may be left unstructured.

COMBINING DIFFERENT LEARNING THEORIES

It is important to point out that learning theories are not mutually exclusive, and you do not have choose only one of these theories to use when designing SBE programmes. Rather, learning theories are complementary. Depending on the SBE programme you are delivering, you may draw upon either single or multiple learning theories. As discussed at the beginning of this chapter, learning theories are frameworks to guide the design of the education. There is nothing incorrect about drawing upon a number of these frameworks, or taking aspects of different theories to guide SBE. An example of an approach to learning that draws upon multiple learning theories is simulation-based mastery learning.

SIMULATION-BASED MASTERY LEARNING

Simulation-based mastery learning is an especially stringent form of competency-based education where learners acquire essential knowledge and skills are measured rigorously against achievement standards (McGaghie et al., 2011a, 2011b). This methodology draws upon behavioural, constructivist, and social cognitive learning theories (McGaghie et al., 2020). It could also be argued that it is also consistent with adult learning theory. The goal of mastery learning is for the learner to 'master' the task/procedure – as opposed to only achieving an acceptable minimum standard. The aim of mastery learning is "excellence for all", with limited variability in performance across a group of learners (McGaghie et al., 2020). Thus, the learning outcomes are uniform for all learners. However, it is recognised that the time taken to achieve these learning outcomes may vary between learners. This approach contrasts with the traditional time-based model of the training of healthcare professionals where the time allowed is often uniform, but the outcomes are variable.

There are seven feature of mastery training:

1. there is baseline testing of performance prior to the commencement of mastery training;
2. there are clear learning objectives in a sequence of units increasing in difficulty;
3. the learner must actively engage in educational activities that are designed to address the learning objectives (e.g., deliberate practice);
4. there is a set minimum passing standard for each educational unit (e.g., test score, number of steps in a procedure performed correctly);
5. the educational units include formative assessment, with feedback;
6. the learner only advances to the next education unit once they have reached, or exceeded, the minimum passing standard; and
7. learners are supported to continue practice or study of an educational unit until the minimum passing standard has been achieved.

(McGaghie et al., 2020)

There is a large body of research on the effectiveness of mastery learning (McGaghie et al., 2014), including evidence of positive effects on patient outcomes (e.g., reduced hospital length of stay, fewer blood transfusions and fewer ICU admissions (Barsuk et al., 2018; see Example 2.4), and other effects such as cost saving (e.g., Cohen et al., 2010)).

The extent to which mastery training draws upon different learning theories is somewhat dependent on what is being taught. To illustrate, if we wished to teach basic clinical procedural skills (e.g., arterial blood gas sampling) using simulation-based mastery training, behavioural learning theory is likely to be the most relevant theory. However, McGaghie et al. (2020) used the example of teaching advanced cardiac life support (ACLS) using simulation-based mastery training to illustrate how multiple learning theories are relevant to teaching the complex set of skills required for ACLS with a simulation-based mastery learning approach. Below is an illustrative example of how four different learning theories can be applied to this complex learning task.

EXAMPLE 2.4   APPLICATION OF MASTERY TRAINING AND SIMULATION

In this study, doctors in training were randomised into a control group that received teaching as usual in how to perform a thoracentesis (a procedure to remove fluid from around the lungs), or a group that received SBE with mastery training to perform the procedure (Barsuk et al., 2018). During the study, 917 thoracenteses were performed on 709 patients. Complication rates for both groups were recorded. It was found that the group that received SBE with mastery training performed thoracenteses with lower rates of clinically meaningful complications than the control group (Barsuk et al., 2018).

- *Adult learning theory.* The learning of ACLS requires a motivated and self-directed learner – one of the tenants of adult learning theory.
- *Behavioural learning theory.* ACLS involves the learning of many specific procedures (e.g., establishing an airway, using a defibrillator). Teaching these skills necessitates the identification of the behaviours that must be performed to complete these procedures, and the conditions under which these behaviours must be performed. These are tenants of behavioural learning theory.
- *Social cognitive learning theory.* ACLS is carried out by a multi-disciplinary team of healthcare professionals. A learner may start by performing one of the more well-defined roles of ACLS (e.g., delivering chest compressions), then rotate through different roles in the arrest team in order to gain confidence and experience before they become the arrest team leader. This approach gives the learner the self-efficacy that they can be a successful team leader – a tenant of social cognitive learning theory.
- *Constructivist learning theory.* Other activities required to successfully deliver ACLS include the ability to recognise, discriminate, and interpret clinical signs and symptoms. The most effective way to obtain these abilities is 'by doing' – a tenant of a constructivist learning theory.

CONCLUSION

We have introduced some of the main learning theories that we believe are particularly relevant to SBE. We hope that we have demonstrated why, and how, learning theories are useful in the design and delivery of SBE. It may be that you naturally gravitate to one theory over another. However, we encourage you to consider what can be taken from a range of learning theories when designing a new SBE programme. We do not suggest starting the design of SBE with a learning theory. Rather, you should identify what you wish to teach, and *then* identify the theory (or combination of theories) that are most appropriate to support the development of a SBE programme.

FURTHER READING

Kaufman, D. M. (2003). ABC of learning and teaching in medicine. *British Medical Journal, 326,* 213–216.
McGaghie, W. C., Harris, I. B. (2018). Learning theory foundations of simulation-based mastery learning. *Simulation in Healthcare, 13*(3S), S15–S20.
Reid-McDermott, B., O'Connor, P., Carey, C., … Byrne, D. (2022). *A Compendium of the Steps Required to Complete 13 Essential Procedural Skills.* The Irish Centre for Applied Patient Safety and Simulation. Galway, Ireland: University of Galway. http://hdl.handle.net/10379/17343
Torre, D. M., Daley, B. J., Sebastian, J. L., Elnicki, D. M. (2006). Overview of current learning theories for medical educators. *American Journal of Medicine, 119*(10), 903–907.

REFERENCES

Ahmed, R., Weaver, L., Falvo, L., Bona, A., Poore, J., Schroedle, K., … Hobgood, C. (2020). Rapid-cycle deliberate practice, death notification. *Clinical Teacher, 17*(6), 644–649.
Artino Jr, A. R., Konopasky, A. (2018). The practical value of educational theory for learning and teaching in graduate medical education. *Journal of Graduate Medicine, 10,* 609–613.
Bandura, A. (1977). *Social Learning Theory.* Englewood Cliffs, NJ: Prentice Hall.
Bandura, A. (1986). *Social Foundations of Thought and Action: A Social Cognitive Theory.* Englewood Cliffs, NJ: Prentice Hall.
Barsuk, J. H., Cohen, E. R., Williams, M. V., Scher, J., Jones, S. F., Feinglass, J., … Wayne, D. B. (2018). Simulation-based mastery learning for thoracentesis skills improves patient outcomes, a randomized trial. *Academic Medicine, 93*(5), 729–735.
Binder, C. (1996). Behavioral fluency, evolution of a new paradigm. *The Behavior Analyst, 19*(2), 163–197.

Chancey, R. J., Sampayo, E. M., Lemke, D. S., Doughty, C. B. (2019). Learners' experiences during rapid cycle deliberate practice simulations, a qualitative analysis. *Simulation in Healthcare*, 14(1), 18–28.

Cohen, E. R., Feinglass, J., Barsuk, J. H., Barnard, C., O'Donnell, A., McGaghie, W. C., Wayne, D. B. (2010). Cost savings from reduced catheter-related bloodstream infection after simulation-based education for residents in a medical intensive care unit. *Simulation in Healthcare*, 5(2), 98–102.

Ericsson, K. A. (2013). Training history, deliberate practice and elite sports performance, an analysis in response to Tucker and Collins review - what makes champions? *British Journal of Sports Medicine*, 47, 533–535.

Ericsson, K. A., Krampe, R. T., Tesch-Römer, C. (1993). The role of deliberate practice in the acquisition of expert performance. *Psychological Review*, 100(3), 363–406.

Gladwell, M. (2008). *Outliers, The Story of Success*. Boston, MA: Little, Brown & Co.

Kaufman, D. M. (2003). Applying educational theory in practice. *BMJ*, 326(7382), 213–216.

Kirwan, B., Ainsworth, L. (1992). *A Guide to Task Analysis*. Boca Raton, FL: CRC Press.

Kolb, D. A. (1984). *Experiential Learning*. Upper Saddle River, NJ: Prentice Hall.

Kubina, R. M., Yurich, K. K. L. (2012). *The Precision Teaching Book*. Lemont, PA: Greatness Achieved Publishing Company.

Lavelle, A., White, M., Griffiths, M., Byrne, D., O'Connor, P. (2020). Human reliability analysis of bronchoscope assisted percutaneous dilatational tracheostomy, implications for simulation based education. *Advances in Simulation*, 5. https://doi.org/10.1186/s41077-020-00149-7

Lydon, S., Burns, N., Healy, O., O'Connor, P., McDermott, B. R., Byrne, D. (2017). Preliminary evaluation of the efficacy of an intervention incorporating precision teaching to train procedural skills among final cycle medical students. *BMJ Simulation & Technology Enhanced Learning*, 3(3), 116.

McGaghie, W. C., Harris, I. B. (2018). Learning theory foundations of simulation-based mastery learning. *Simulation in Healthcare*, 13(3S), S15–S20.

McGaghie, W. C., Issenberg, S. B., Barsuk, J. H., Wayne, D. B. (2014). A critical review of simulation-based mastery learning with translational outcomes. *Medical Education*, 48(4), 375–385.

McGaghie, W. C., Issenberg, S. B., Cohen, E. R., Barsuk, J. H., Wayne, B. (2011a). Does simulation-based medical education with deliberate practice yield better results than traditional clinical education? A meta-analytic comparative review of the evidence. *Academic Medicine*, 86(6), 706–711.

McGaghie, W. C., Issenberg, S. B., Cohen, E. R., Barsuk, J. H., Wayne, D. B. (2011b). Medical education featuring mastery learning with deliberate practice can lead to better health for individuals and populations. *Academic Medicine*, 86(11), e8–e9.

McGaghie, W. C., Wayne, D. B., Barsuk, J. H. (2020). Translational science and healthcare quality and safety improvement from mastery learning. In C. McGagfhie, J.H. Barsuk, D.B. Wayne (Eds.), *Comprehensive Healthcare Simulation, Mastery Learning in Health Professions Education* (pp. 289–307). Berlin: Springer.

McGaghie, W. C., Wayne, D. B., Barsuk, J. H., Issenberg, S. B. (2021). Deliberate practice and mastery learning contributions to medical education and improved healthcare. *Journal of Expertise*, 4(2), 144–168.

Reddy, K., Byrne, D., Breen, D., Lydon, S., O'Connor, P. (2020). The application of human reliability analysis to three critical care procedures. *Reliability Engineering and System Safety*, 203,107–116.

Reid-McDermott, B., O'Connor, P., Carey, C., … Byrne, D. (2022). *A Compendium of the Steps Required to Complete 13 Essential Procedural Skills*. The Irish Centre for Applied Patient Safety and Simulation. Galway, Ireland: University of Galway.

Rosman, S. L., Nyirasafari, R., Bwiza, H. M., Umuhoza, C., Camp, E. A., Weiner, D. L., Rus, M. C. (2019). Rapid cycle deliberate practice vs. traditional simulation in a resource-limited setting. *BMC Medical Education*, 19(1), 1–8.

Rourke, L., Schmidt, M., Garga, N. (2010). Theory-based research of high fidelity simulation use in nursing education, a review of the literature. *International Journal of Nursing Education Scholarship*, 7(1).

Torre, D. M., Daley, B. J., Sebastian, J. L., Elnicki, D. M. (2006). Overview of current learning theories for medical educators. *American Journal of Medicine*, 119(10), 903–907.

Zigmont, J. J., Kappus, L. J., Sudikoff, S. N. (2011). Theoretical foundations of learning through simulation. *Seminars in Perinatology*, 35(2), 47–51.

3 Instructional Design

KEY POINTS

- The goal of instructional design is to construct a programme of instruction that optimises the learning for participants.
- The ADDIE (Analyse, Design, Develop, Implement, and Evaluate) model is one of the common approaches for instructional design.
- Learning outcomes are broad in scope, and related to the whole simulation-based education (SBE) activity. In contrast, learning objectives are specific and detailed and relate to specific knowledge, skills, and attitudes.
- When designing SBE, we recommend first identifying the overall learning outcomes, and then from these deriving the learning objectives for the simulation scenario.
- Evaluation of SBE can be considered at a number of levels: (1) reactions (did the learners like it?); (2) learning (did the learners increase their knowledge or change their attitudes?); (3) behaviour (did the learners change their behaviour?); (4) results (was there an impact on patient care?); and (5) return-on-investment (did the programme save money?).

INTRODUCTION

Instructional design can be defined as "the principles and procedures by which instructional, materials, lessons, and whole systems can be developed in a consistent and reliable fashion" (Molenda et al., 2003: 52). Instructional design is concerned with the comprehensive process of developing instruction from beginning to end. Instructional design requires a proper design process in which the educational needs of the learners are identified, training is designed to meet these needs, and an evaluation as to whether these needs have been met by the learners. The goal of instructional design is to construct a programme of instruction that optimises the learning for participants.

CHAPTER OUTLINE

This chapter will describe the Analyse, Design, Develop, Implement, and Evaluate (ADDIE) model of instructional design and outline how the model can be applied to the development of simulation-based education (SBE) programmes. In addition, this chapter will discuss the design of training evaluation, and how to assess the return-on-investment of training interventions.

THE ADDIE MODEL

There are many different approaches to designing, developing, and delivering training or education. The ADDIE model is the most common, and even if it is not specifically used, it forms the foundation of other models of instructional design. The ADDIE model is so pervasive it has been described as being virtually synonymous with instructional systems development (Molenda et al., 2003). The origins and developers of the ADDIE model are not entirely clear. What is known is that the model was first conceived in the mid-1970s through a collaboration between Florida State University and the US Department of Defense (Molenda, 2003). The ADDIE acronym stands for the

DOI: 10.1201/9781003296942-3

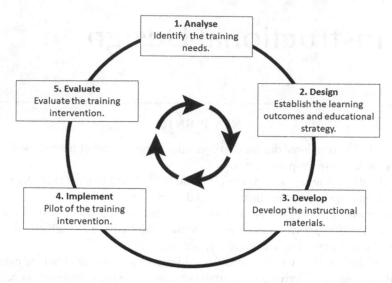

FIGURE 3.1   The ADDIE model.

five stages of the model: Analyse, Design, Develop, Implement, and Evaluate (see Figure 3.1). Each stage of the ADDIE model will be described in more detail below.

STAGE 1: ANALYSE

This first stage of the ADDIE model is concerned with identifying what you need to teach. This is commonly described as a training needs assessment. The analysis stage is crucial, but it is an easy stage to either ignore or fail to complete adequately. A good training needs assessment will pay dividends when it comes to designing SBE (see Example 3.1 (analyse) for an overview of the analyse stage of a training programme that used the ADDIE model). There is little point in developing a training or educational programme that does not address the needs of the learners, and ultimately

---

EXAMPLE 3.1   ANALYSE

The analysis of high-profile adverse events in healthcare suggests that junior doctors often do not raise concerns or 'speak up' when circumstance demands it. Therefore, a need was identified for a training intervention that teaches junior doctors to speak up. The target population was newly graduated medical students in the first year of clinical practice, (known in Ireland as interns). Three sources of information were scrutinised in order to identify the training needs of this group.

1. A review of research evidence exploring the causes of poor speaking-up behaviour in junior doctors.
2. A literature review of existing training interventions designed to support communication and teamwork in healthcare and other high-risk domains such as aviation.
3. The analysis of the performance of junior doctors in a series of five human factors–focused standardised patient scenarios.

The analysis phase culminated in the identification of core skills and attitudes related to assertiveness and communication, which are needed but often lacking in junior doctors (O'Connor et al., 2013).

the needs of the organisation. Failing to meet these needs means the opportunity for developing a worthwhile training programme is lost.

Ideas for training often come from the clinical environment where deficiencies in skill have been identified, or from training bodies that have identified the competencies expected at various stages of training. Irrespective of the origin of the training need, a training needs analysis should be conducted in order to ensure that all the aspects of the required skill or competency is fully understood. Clearly, there will be constraints on how extensive the training needs analysis might be (e.g., availability of resources). Moreover, in most cases it will not be feasible, nor necessary, to do a big analysis project in order to identify the training needs. However, it is suggested that at a minimum a literature review would be beneficial to investigate what has been written on the subject, and to identify whether there are other education or training approaches that you could use or adapt.

It is also important to talk to people who perform, and perhaps observe, whatever you are interested in training. If you are interested in teaching a particular clinical procedural skill, you might see if you can find an existing task analysis (see Chapter 2 for a discussion) outlining the steps in the procedure, talking to people who perform the procedure on a regular basis, and watching them perform the procedure in either an actual, or simulated, environment. For example, the procedure shown below (see Example 3.2) on how to perform a 12-lead electrocardiogram was developed by a paramedic and ICU nurse who are experienced in carrying out this procedure.

EXAMPLE 3.2   STEPS REQUIRED TO PERFORM A 12-LEAD ELECTROCARDIOGRAM

Prepare consumables/equipment

1. Perform hand hygiene.
2. Clean ECG machine.

Prepare self

3. Perform hand hygiene.

Prepare patient

4. Position the patient.
5. Expose the patient.
6. Prepare the patient's skin.
7. Remove non-sterile gloves.
8. Perform hand hygiene.
9. Identify anatomical landmark.

During procedure

10. Prepare the ECG adhesive electrode.
11–20. Place CHEST electrodes on the patient in the appropriate place in the order: V1; V2; V4; V3; V5; V6; RA (red); LA (yellow); RL (black); and LL (green).
21. Attach ECG cables to the electrodes on the patient.
22. Enter the patient details into ECG machine.
23. Perform final checks before performing ECG.
24. Perform the ECG.
25. Turn off the ECG machine.
26. Remove the ECG cables.
27. Remove ECG electrodes from the patient.

Clean up

28. Clean the ECG machine and return to its charging station.
29. Dispose of all waste.
30. Perform hand hygiene.

(adapted from Reid-McDermott et al., 2022)

STAGE 2: DESIGN

In the design stage the skills and knowledge identified through the needs analysis are transformed into learning outcomes/objectives and a training strategy (Der Sahakian et al., 2019).

LEARNING OUTCOMES AND LEARNING OBJECTIVES

Learning outcomes and learning objectives are closely related concepts in education. They are often used interchangeably and, in fact, whether the differences matters has been questioned (Prideaux, 2000). Nonetheless, we believe that the distinction is important in instructional design. Harden (2002) provides some useful guidance on the distinction between the two concepts. Outcomes are broad in scope, and related to the whole SBE activity. For example: "on completion of the simulation activity the learner will be able to identify a deteriorating patient and escalate appropriately". In contrast, learning objectives are specific and detailed and relate to specific knowledge, skills, and attitudes. For example: "the learner will escalate care to an appropriate senior using ISBAR [Introduction, Situation, Background, Assessment and Recommendation]". Learning objectives should be used to design the simulation scenario (see Chapter 4) and the debrief (see Chapter 7). Learning outcomes are intended to be met by the learner. As such, they are particularly important if a summative assessment of the learners is to be carried out (see Chapter 8). In contrast, learning objectives can be viewed as an intended achievement (Harden, 2002). As such, it may be that a particular learner fails to achieve a learning objective (e.g., does not use ISBAR). A final consideration is that Harden (2002) suggests that learning objectives reflect a teacher-centred approach, in which the focus is on what the instructor wants to teach. In contrast, learning outcomes encourage a learner-centred approach in which the teacher considers what it is that the learner should be able to do. As such, when designing SBE, we recommend first identifying the overall learning outcomes, and then from these deriving the learning objectives for the simulation scenario.

A common approach to writing learning outcomes/objectives is to use Bloom's Revised Taxonomy (Chatterjee & Corral, 2017; Der Sahakian et al., 2019; Miller et al., 2021). Blooms' Revised Taxonomy (Krathwohl, 2002) has three domains of learning: (1) cognitive (knowledge); (2) skills (psychomotor); and (3) affective (attitudes). The taxonomy has a hierarchy of six levels from 'remember' to 'create' (see Figure 3.2). It is possible to align these levels to different SBE learning activities. It is certainly not necessary to have learning outcomes/objectives associated with every level. However, as can be seen in Figure 3.2, the taxonomy is useful in thinking about considering how to design learning outcomes/objectives.

Rudolf et al. (2008) made the following recommendations for writing effective learning objectives. They should be:

- *Specific*: the learning objective is specific and focused with a clear outline of what the learner is expected to achieve with an appropriate active verb (see Figure 3.2 for examples of some verbs).

- *Observable*: whether the objective has been achieved should be clearly perceptible.
- *Achievable*: it is reasonable to expect the target learners to achieve the objective.
- *Appropriate*: the learning objective is realistic and can be achieved given the resources and time available for the teaching activity.
- *Easy to assess*: an assessment can be made of whether the learning objective has been achieved.

For example, 'the learner will demonstrate closed loop communication'; or 'the learner will follow the sepsis 6 pathway'.

TEACHING STRATEGY

The learning outcomes/objectives inform which learning theory (or combination of theories) should form the foundation of the training (see Chapter 2). The theoretical foundation will then inform which strategy of training is appropriate. Decisions on the teaching strategy will also be informed by the most effective and efficient approach to meeting the learning outcomes/objectives. It may become apparent that a particular learning outcome/objective cannot be achieved with the resources available (e.g., Example 3.3: Design). In which case, there is a need to either change the learning outcome/objective or increase the resources. The design phase will culminate in the identification of methods and modalities that will be employed in the training, taking practicality, time, and space limitations into consideration.

There is a need to consider which simulation modality is most appropriate to use in order to support the achievement of the learning outcome/objective. If the learning outcome/objective are focused on the lower levels of Bloom's Revised Taxonomy (i.e., remembering or understanding; see Figure 3.2), it may be that a more traditional classroom-based approach is a more efficient and cost-effective approach to teaching than SBE. SBE is most appropriate for the middle four levels of the taxonomy (see Figure 3.2). However, there is still a need to consider which is the most appropriate simulation modality to meet each learning outcome/objective (see Chapter 1 for an overview of the different modalities).

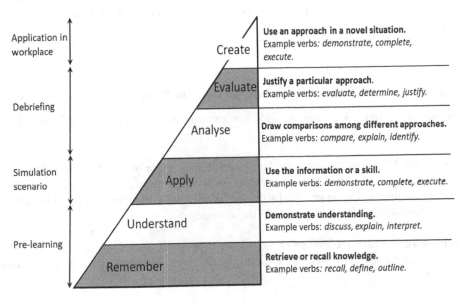

FIGURE 3.2 Alignment between Bloom's Revised Taxonomy (Krathwohl, 2002) and SBE activities.

EXAMPLE 3.3 DESIGN (Continues on from the Analysis Stage Described Above)

Learning outcome: The interns will be able to speak up when they have a patient safety concern.

Learning objectives: On completion of the training, the interns will be able to:

1. explain why speaking up is important for patient safety;
2. demonstrate a range of practical strategies to enhance communication in healthcare settings; and
3. apply specific communication strategies in appropriate situations.

Training methods: There was 90 minutes available to deliver the training. Therefore, it was decided that it was not feasible to design a simulation-based training programme – although the training would support other simulation-based training provided to the participants. The theoretical foundation of the training was based upon experiential learning theory (see Chapter 2). The training was also modelled on an approach that is often used in aviation in which filmed re-enactments are used to demonstrate examples of good and poor performance (Flin et al., 2008). It was too difficult and costly to produce re-enactments of medical mishaps. Therefore, it was decided to conduct recorded interviews with senior doctors, describing a challenging event they had been involved in where speaking up or lack of speaking up was a factor in the event. To facilitate discussion, a small-group teaching method for the programme was planned (O'Connor et al., 2013).

STAGE 3: DEVELOP

Once the learning outcomes/objectives, appropriate learning theory, and the teaching strategy have been identified, the next stage of the ADDIE model is to develop all of the instructional materials required to deliver the SBE intervention (see Example 3.4). These materials might include: lesson plans, instructional content, simulation scenarios, and assessment tools. Scenario development is discussed in detail in the next chapter. It is important to consider all of the requirements to deliver the training. These may include:

EXAMPLE 3.4 DEVELOP (Continues On from the Design Stage Described Above)

Instructional content: A 20-minute slide presentation was developed by a human factors psychologist that:

1. introduced the concept of human factors and human error in healthcare;
2. identified and described the non-technical skills required of an effective intern; and
3. provided instruction on practical strategies to enhance communication (see Brindley and Reynolds (2011) for a review of these strategies).

Video resources: Video-recordings of interviews with senior doctors were produced for use within the training session. These were used to generate small-group discussions (O'Connor et al., 2013).

- *Resources* – is there a need for specific equipment or consumables?
- *Personnel* – who is required to deliver the training? – Instructors, simulation technicians, other personnel that may be required (e.g., standardised participants)
- *Learners* – how many learners are to be trained at once? When are the learners available to attend the training?
- *Scheduling* – when and where will the training take place? Are suitable facilities with the required equipment (e.g., audio-visual equipment) available? Are the facilities available for when the training is planned to be delivered?

STAGE 4: IMPLEMENT

In this fourth stage a pilot of the actual SBE intervention as it is intended to be run, is completed. In research, a pilot study is defined as "a study in which a future study or part of a future study, is conducted on a smaller scale to ask the question whether something can be done, should we proceed with it, and if so, how" (Eldridge et al., 2016: 8). The purpose of a pilot of a SBE intervention is similar to that of a pilot research study. This pilot training should be completed in a way that is as close as possible to what is planned in terms of the content, the schedule, the facilities, and the learner. The purpose of the pilot training is to identify any unanticipated issues, errors, or problems. If problems are identified, it may be necessary to return to one of the earlier stages in the ADDIE model in order to make changes, and then complete another pilot. As with the analysis phase, the extent to which the SBE intervention is piloted will be dependent on the resources that are available. However, at a minimum, any new training should be piloted at least once, or more often if large issues were identified (see Example 3.5).

Designing and piloting the SBE interventions are crucial. What is often more difficult is the process of integrating the training intervention into an existing curriculum and sustaining the intervention in the long term. Ideally, training will be sustainable, without any overreliance on those who initially developed the programme. Utilisation of the principles of implementation science can support this integration process. Implementation science is defined as "the study of methods to promote the systematic uptake of evidence-based programmes and practices into a health setting and thus to improve the quality and effectiveness of intervention delivery" (Eccles & Mittman, 2006: 1). An implementation science approach is systematic and is concerned with the design, refinement, evaluation, and implementation of SBE and aims to take the complexity of the training context into consideration. Full consideration of implementation science is beyond the scope of this chapter but those interested in finding out more should look at the Haji et al. (2014) and Price et al. (2015) papers in the recommended further readings at the end of this chapter. Example 3.6 demonstrates how issues with implementation can negatively impact SBE.

EXAMPLE 3.5   IMPLEMENT (Continues On from the Develop Stage Described Above)

Pilot implementation: The study was piloted with a group of six staff members with a background in either medicine or human factors. Based on this pilot, the number of slides in the presentation was reduced, and one of the four videos was dropped. The main rationale for this change was to foster more conversation from the participants, and ensure the training could be completed within 90 minutes.

Full implementation: A total of 110 interns in a training hospital attended the training in groups of between 6 and 12 learners. The training was delivered by a human factors psychologist in a small classroom with a computer, screen, and audio speakers (O'Connor et al., 2013).

> ## EXAMPLE 3.6   EVALUATION OF THE IMPACT OF SIMULATION-BASED TRAINING ON PATIENT OUTCOMES (LENGUERRAND ET AL., 2020)
>
> The Practical Obstetrics Multi-Professional Training package (PROMPT) is a simulation-based training programme that covers the management of obstetric emergencies. Single-site assessments of the training demonstrated improved compliance with clinical standards, reductions in clinical error, and sustainable improvements in perinatal outcomes (Lenguerrand et al., 2020).
>
> The aim of the study was to deliver PROMPT across 12 large maternity hospitals with the aim of reducing the proportion of term babies with an Apgar score $<7^{5mins}$. A two-day training programme was provided on how to deliver PROMPT at each hospital. The PROMPT training was then delivered at each unit. The goal was to train all staff within a 12-month period.
>
> The intervention did not lead to a reduction in the proportion of term babies with an Apgar score $<7^{5mins}$ (1.32% pre-intervention to 1.59% post-intervention). The lack of an effect was attributed to issues with implementation rather than the intervention itself. There was considerable variability in the implementation across units. For example, there were delays in starting the training in some units, and there was no funding to support data collection by staff at some units so the proportion of staff trained could not be derived. Additionally, simultaneous, and sometimes contradictory, national training programmes were also introduced during the period of the intervention which may have contaminated the effects of the study.

STAGE 5: EVALUATE

This final stage of the ADDIE model of instructional design is concerned with evaluating the SBE intervention. This stage requires a consideration of what should be evaluated, and when the evaluation should take place. A commonly used approach to considering how to evaluate education and training programmes is Kirkpatrick's (1998) four-level model: (1) reactions; (2) learning; (3) behaviour; and (4) results. Philips (2003) also added a fifth level of return-on-investment (see Example 3.7).

Level 1: Reactions. Reactions are concerned with assessing what the learners thought about the SBE intervention – Did they like it?, Did they think it was useful?, etc. These are often paper and pencil questionnaires completed immediately after the programme is completed. These are general short questionnaires with a mix of Likert-scale questions (e.g., "the learning outcomes of the training was clear, please respond from (1) very unclear, to (5) very clear"), and open-ended questions (e.g., "How could the training be improved?"). It is important to indicate positive reaction does not ensure learning. Although, a negative reaction almost certainly reduces the likelihood that this has taken place (Kirkpatrick, 1998).

Level 2: Learning (attitudes and knowledge). Learning refers to "the principles, facts, and skills which were understood and absorbed by the participants" (Kirkpatrick, 1976: 11). At this level, an assessment is made as to whether the learners have either gained knowledge, or have changed their attitudes or beliefs as a result of the SBE intervention. Attitudes are commonly assessed using a questionnaire. It is preferable to use an existing attitudes questionnaire rather than creating a new one. However, it is important that the questionnaire matches with the learning objectives. It is also possible to assess attitudes more qualitatively using an interview approach. A knowledge assessment can be readily carried out using multiple choice, or short answer questions. However, it is important that the assessment is consistent with the learning objectives and the content of the SBE intervention.

Level 3: Behaviour. For SBE interventions, behaviour is arguably the most important assessment as the focus of this type of training is on teaching behaviours. Therefore, an assessment of whether

EXAMPLE 3.7   EVALUATE (Continues On from the Implement Stage Described Above)

An evaluation was carried out at the first three levels of Kirkpatrick's evaluation hierarchy.

1. *Reactions.* A nine-item reactions questionnaire was designed to collect information on what the participants thought about the training, and whether they found it interesting, useful, and, relevant.
2. *Learning (attitudes and knowledge).* Knowledge was assessed using a combination of multiple-choice and open-ended questions, derived from the content of the training. Attitudes were assessed using two scales (12 items) from a questionnaire designed to assess attitudes to speaking up (O'Connor, et al., 2012).
3. *Behaviour.* Behaviour was assessed using a pre-post study design using two simulated participant scenarios (one pre- and one post-). The sample consisted of 50 interns who had participated in the training, and 35 interns from a control group who had not participated in the training (O'Connor et al., 2013). In each scenario, participants were required to demonstrate the skills and attitudes that were targeted in the training session. The interns were observed using a rating form specifically designed for each scenario.

Outcome. The reactions from the learners was positive. There was a significant increase in knowledge as a result of the training, and some evidence to support a shift in attitudes in the desirable direction relating to the need to speak up to seniors. However, no effect of the training was found on behaviour. This training has continued to be delivered each year to >100 interns annually.

these skills or behaviours have improved is an important consideration. Summative and formative assessment of behaviour are discussed in detail in Chapter 8.

Level 4: Results. The ultimate aim of any SBE intervention is to produce tangible evidence of an impact at "organisational" level. In the context of healthcare, this is generally considered to translate to showing an impact on patient care or patient outcomes. Examples of the impact of a SBE intervention on patient care include improved time-based targets in trauma (Härgestam et al., 2016) and strokes (Ajmi et al., 2019), and improved resuscitation outcomes (Josey et al., 2018). Evaluating the impact of SBE on patient outcomes is more challenging than for the other levels of Kirkpatrick's (1998) evaluation hierarchy. It may also be difficult to establish suitable organisational-level measures that directly relate to a SBE intervention. Therefore, it could be that there is a lack of an effect at the organisational level, not because the intervention is ineffective, but because the measure of the organisational effect of the SBE is modulated by a range of other factors that are unrelated to the intervention (e.g., issues with implementation – see Example 3.6).

Level 5: Return-on-Investment (ROI). The purpose of the ROI assessment is to establish if the monetary value of the results of SBE exceeded the cost of delivering the intervention. Despite the potential benefits associated with a cost analysis of SBE interventions, such assessments are rarely reported in the research literature (Hippe et al., 2020). However, due to the expense of SBE there is arguably increasing pressure to demonstrate the value of this approach (Hippe et al., 2020). Philips (2003) provides some guidance on how to assess the ROI of SBE interventions.

- *Assess training impact.* Firstly, there is a need to assess the impact of the training by evaluating at one or more of the levels of Kirkpatrick's (1998) evaluation hierarchy and assessing the impact of the SBE intervention (see below for a discussion of different designs for assessing the effectiveness of educational programmes). Theilen et al. (2017) described an assessment of a weekly paediatric in situ simulation training intervention designed to improve the performance of emergency teams. In terms of the ROI, an assessment was made of whether there was a change in the number of paediatric intensive care unit (PICU) bed days associated with unplanned admissions from deteriorating ward patients.

- *Isolate the training effect.* This is concerned with assessing the impact of only the SBE intervention. For Theilen et al. (2017), the training effect was the number of PICU bed days associated with unplanned admissions from deteriorating ward patients. In the year prior to the training intervention there were 527 associated PICU bed days. Three years after the introduction of the training intervention there was 193 associated PICU bed days.

- *Monetising the training effects.* To carry out a ROI, the training effect must be converted into a monetary value. Theilen et al. (2017) used an estimate of £2,400 for a PICU bed day. Prior to the training intervention the cost of the associated PICU bed days was £1,264,800 (£2,400 multiplied by 527). Three years after the introduction of the training intervention the cost of the associated PICU bed days was £463,200 (£2,400 multiplied by 193). Therefore, the training intervention resulted in a saving of £801,600 (£1,264,800 minus £463,200).

- *Estimate the cost of delivering the SBE intervention.* When estimating the cost of delivery of the training, all costs should be included. Theilen et al. (2017) calculated a cost of £74,250 per annum to deliver the training intervention. The cost for the training included: scenario development, delivery of 48 two-hour training sessions, staff meetings, faculty meetings, review of relevant calls and unplanned admissions, protected training time for attendees, consumables and maintenance of manikins. This resulted in a total estimated cost of £74,250 per annum to deliver the training. Theilen et al. (2017) also indicated that there were 'sunk costs' (i.e., a cost that has already been incurred and that cannot be recovered) to buy a medium-fidelity paediatric manikin, monitor and tablet. Generally, sunk costs are not included in the calculation of the ROI.

- *Return-on-investment (ROI) calculation.* Once the benefits and costs of delivering the SBE intervention have been calculated, the following formula can then be used to calculate the ROI (Bukhari et al., 2017).

$$ROI(\%) = \frac{\text{Net benefit of SBE intervention}}{\text{Cost of delivering SBE intervention}} \times 100$$

So, for the Theilen et al. (2017) training intervention the ROI was:

$$\frac{£801,600}{£74,250} \times 100 = 1,079\%.$$

This ROI provides very strong evidence of the ROI of the training intervention.

New World Kirkpatrick Model

Reviews of the use of Kirkpatrick's evaluation hierarchy reveal that most investigators in medical education do not evaluate beyond the learning level (Yardley & Dornan, 2012). A suggested reason for this is that people run out of evaluation resources or motivation after completing an evaluation of reaction and learning (Moreau, 2017). To address some of the issues with the evaluation hierarchy, there has been a revision developed called the New World Kirkpatrick Model (NWKM; Kirkpatrick & Kirkpatrick, 2016). The NWKM is closely aligned to the original Kirkpatrick's hierarchy of evaluation, with a few key changes and recommendations. Firstly, in the NWKM model the levels of evaluation have been reversed, i.e., result is level 1, and reactions is level 4. The rationale for this reversal is to encourage a design and an evaluation with a focus on the main outcome of the training, e.g., improve patient safety. Also, Kirkpatrick and Kirkpatrick (2016) make the point that it may not be necessary to evaluate at every level of the hierarchy, so consideration should be given to ensuring that the most important or meaningful evaluations are performed. In the case of SBE interventions this is likely to include behaviour. It is also recommended that the evaluation should be embedded and a planned part of instructional design process, rather than added as an afterthought (Kirkpatrick & Kirkpatrick, 2016). Finally, the NWKM recognises the impact that learner characteristics (e.g., motivation) and organisational factors (e.g., reinforcement of desirable behaviours) can have on evaluation outcomes.

TRAINING EVALUATION DESIGNS

Consistent with Kirkpatrick and Kirkpatrick's (2016) recommendation to include the evaluation as part of the instructional design, in addition to deciding what to evaluate, it is also important to consider when the evaluation should be carried out. Figure 3.3 provides an overview of common approaches to instructional design, each with an increasing level of rigour (but also complexity to achieve) from design 1 to design 3.

The first design shown in Figure 3.3 is a post-test-only design. In this design, evaluation is only carried out after the training has occurred and there is no control group. As such, it is not possible to assess whether there has been a change as a result of the training. Therefore, this approach is most applicable to the collection of reactions-level data on what learners thought about the training.

The second design in Figure 3.3 is a pre-test post-test design. As there is a pre-training assessment, it is possible to make a comparison of the impact of the training. This comparison is often done immediately after the training. However, a meta-analysis of skill decay has found that if the skill is not either used or practiced in a year, there is a large decay in performance (one standard

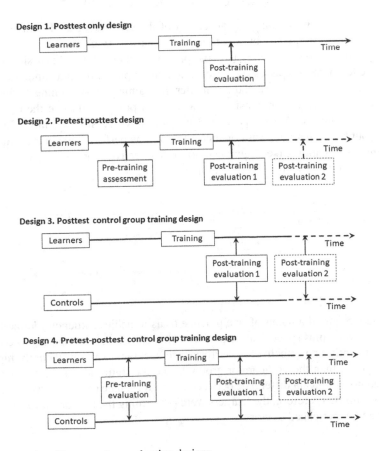

FIGURE 3.3 Educational intervention evaluation designs.

deviation), and cognitive skills decay more quickly than psychomotor skills (Arthur et al., 1998). Therefore, it might be worth considering an additional evaluation beyond an immediate assessment of effectiveness. Moreover, a pre-test post-test design does not utilise a control group and as such it does not control for the effect of history (i.e., effects of events that can happen at the same time as the training that may influence the outcomes). It may also be the evaluation itself has an impact (e.g., if the learners are given the same knowledge test before and after the training they may improve their performance as they have seen the test before).

In the third design in Figure 3.3 (post-test-only control group design) a comparison is made with a control group that has not participated in the training. The main advantages of this design, as compared to design 2, is that it controls for the effect of history and the effect of the evaluation. So, for example, if there was a change in procedures implemented after post-training 1 that may impact the evaluation, this would be addressed in design 3 as there is a control group who completes the evaluation at the same time as the intervention group.

Design 4 is the most rigorous of the designs in Figure 3.3. This design is a combination of designs 2 and 3. However, design 4 requires more resources to carry out than the other designs. Example 3.8 describes a study that uses aspects of both designs 3 and 4 to evaluate the effect of a precision teaching intervention.

The design of any evaluation should be carefully considered. It is not necessary, nor perhaps possible, to always complete a rigorous evaluation of a training course. In the research literature, a

---

EXAMPLE 3.8   EXAMPLE EVALUATION OF THE IMPACT OF PRECISION TEACHING (LYDON ET AL., 2019)

In this pilot study an evaluation was carried out of the efficacy of a SBE intervention. The intervention involved frequency building and precision teaching strategies for training lumbar puncture to behavioural fluency (see the previous chapter for a discussion of precision teaching). The learners were assessed performing lumbar puncture on a simulator prior to the training (pre-training evaluation), and again after the training (post-training evaluation 1; see figure below). The intervention consisted of a series of practice trials of the procedure with feedback on performance. A retrospective chart audit of successful and failed lumbar punctures carried out by the learners was conducted to examine performance in the clinical setting. At post-training evaluation 2 (see figure below) a retrospective chart review was carried out of performance of lumbar puncture on real infant patients.

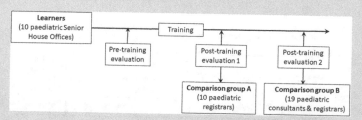

The learners required a mean of five practice trials to achieve fluency (defined as a combination of accuracy plus speed that demonstrate the learners are competent to complete the procedure efficiently and effectively). Performance accuracy was significantly higher in the intervention group than the comparator group A (see the figure above). Retrospective chart audit revealed no significant difference between the performance of the intervention group and comparator group B. Therefore, the learners were performing the task at a level comparable to more senior and experienced doctors.

pre-test post-test design is common. The important point is to consider, and plan for an evaluation design that can be achieved with the resources you have available.

FINAL THOUGHTS ON THE ADDIE MODEL

The ADDIE model provides a useful and practical framework for how to develop a SBE intervention. As presented in this chapter, it may seem very prescriptive and is not possible to move to the next stage of the model until the previous one is completed. However, the reality is that it is unlikely that the development process will be quite as linear as described here, and it may be necessary to move forwards and backwards through the stages. It also may not be necessary to stick rigidly to the stages in the ADDIE model. This is particularly true if a SBE intervention is not being developed from first principles, but is being adapted from an existing training programme. However, there can be a tendency to focus on the design, development, and implementation of the SBE intervention and ignore the analyse and evaluation stages. The risk of ignoring these two stages is that it will then be difficult to identify whether the SBE intervention is meeting the needs of the learner or having the desired effect on performance.

CONCLUSION

The Society for Simulation in Healthcare Research Committee (Anton et al., 2022) identified the research priorities in healthcare simulation as judged by simulation experts. The top three priorities were identified as: (1) evaluating the impact of system-level simulation interventions on system efficiency, patient safety, and patient outcomes; (2) evaluating the ROI of simulation for healthcare systems; and (3) evaluating whether a dose–response relationship exists between simulation training and performance/patient outcomes. These research questions can only be answered through the use of a rigorous approach to instructional design and programme evaluation.

We believe that the ADDIE model and Kirkpatrick's evaluation hierarchy are useful for supporting instructional design. However, it is important to be both pragmatic and realistic in terms of the extent to which we must stick rigidly to the ADDIE model, and the rigour required in the design and the evaluation of the instructional design process. What is necessary to answer the Society for Simulation in Healthcare Research Committee's priorities is not the same as designing and evaluating a small SBE intervention at one hospital.

FURTHER READING

Der Sahakian, G., Buléon, C., Alinier, G. (2019). Educational foundations of instructional design applied to simulation-based education. In Chiniara, G. (Ed.) *Clinical Simulation Education, Operations, and Engineering* (pp 185–206). Amsterdam, Netherlands: Elsevier.

Haji, F. A., Da Silva, C., Daigle, D. T., Dubrowski, A. (2014). From bricks to buildings, adapting the medical research council framework to develop programs of research in simulation education and training for the health professions. *Simulation in Healthcare*, 9(4), 249–259.

Harden, R. M. (2002). Learning outcomes and instructional objectives, is there a difference? *Medical Teacher*, 24(2), 151–155.

INACSL Standards Committee, Miller, C., Deckers, C., Jones, M., Wells-Beede, E., McGee, E. (2021). Healthcare simulation standards of best practice outcomes and objectives. *Clinical Simulation in Nursing*, 58, 40–44.

Peterson, C. (2003). Bringing ADDIE to life, instructional design at its best. *Journal of Educational Multimedia and Hypermedia*, 12(3), 227–241.

Price, D. W., Wagner, D. P., Krane, N. K., Rougas, S. C., Lowitt, N. R., Offodile, R. S., ... Barnes, B. E. (2015). What are the implications of implementation science for medical education? *Medical Education Online*, 20(1), 27003.

Terrell, M. (2006). Anatomy of learning, Instructional design principles for the anatomical sciences. *The Anatomical Record Part B, The New Anatomist*, 289(6), 252–260.

ONLINE RESOURCES

- What is Bloom's Taxonomy?- www.youtube.com/watch?v=fqgTBwElPzU
- Kirkpatrick Partners: www.kirkpatrickpartners.com/. A range of learning materials on Kirkpatrick's evaluation hierarchy.

REFERENCES

Anton, N., Calhoun, A.C., Stefanidis, D. (2022). Current research priorities in healthcare simulation, results of a Delphi survey. *Simulation in Healthcare*, *17*(1), e1–e7.

Ajmi, S. C., Advani, R., Fjetland, L., Kurz, K. D., Lindner, T., Qvindesland, S. A., … Kurz, M. (2019). Reducing door-to-needle times in stroke thrombolysis to 13 min through protocol revision and simulation training, a quality improvement project in a Norwegian stroke centre. *BMJ Quality & Safety*, *28*(11), 939–948.

Arthur Jr, W., Bennett Jr, W., Stanush, P. L., McNelly, T. L. (1998). Factors that influence skill decay and retention, a quantitative review and analysis. *Human Performance*, *11*(1), 57–101.

Brindley, P. G., Reynolds, S. F. (2011). Improving verbal communication in critical care medicine. *Journal of Critical Care*, *26*(2), 155–159.

Bukhari, H., Andreatta, P., Goldiez, B., Rabelo, L. (2017). A framework for determining the return on investment of simulation-based training in health care. *Journal of Health Care Organization, Provision, and Financing*, *54*, 1–7.

Chatterjee, D., Corral, J. (2017). How to write well-defined learning objectives. *Journal of Education in Perioperative Medicine*, *19*(4), e610.

Der Sahakian, G., Buléon, C., Alinier, G. (2019). Educational foundations of instructional design applied to simulation-based education. In Chiniara, G. (Ed.) *Clinical Simulation Education, Operations, and Engineering* (pp 185–206). Amsterdam, Netherlands: Elsevier.

Eccles, M. P., Mittman, B. S. (2006). Welcome to implementation science. *Implementation Science*, *1*(1), 1.

Eldridge, S. M., Lancaster, G. A., Campbell, M. J., Thabane, L., Hopewell, S., Coleman, C. L., Bond, C. M. (2016). Defining feasibility and pilot studies in preparation for randomised controlled trials, development of a conceptual framework. *PloS One*, *11*(3), e0150205.

Flin, R., O'Connor, P., Crichton, M. (2008). *Safety at the Sharp End, Training Non-technical Skills*. Aldershot, UK: Ashgate.

Haji, F. A., Da Silva, C., Daigle, D. T., Dubrowski, A. (2014). From bricks to buildings, adapting the medical research council framework to develop programs of research in simulation education and training for the health professions. *Simulation in Healthcare*, *9*(4), 249–259.

Harden, R. M. (2002). Learning outcomes and instructional objectives, is there a difference? *Medical Teacher*, *24*(2), 151–155.

Härgestam, M., Lindkvist, M., Jacobsson, M., Brulin, C., Hultin, M. (2016). Trauma teams and time to early management during in situ trauma team training. *BMJ Open*, *6*(1), e009911.

Hippe, D. S., Umoren, R. A., McGee, A., Bucher, S. L., Bresnahan, B. W. (2020). A targeted systematic review of cost analyses for implementation of simulation-based education in healthcare. *SAGE Open Medicine*, *8*, 1–9.

Josey, K., Smith, M. L., Kayani, A. S., Young, G., Kasperski, M. D., Farrer, P., … Raschke, R. A. (2018). Hospitals with more-active participation in conducting standardized in-situ mock codes have improved survival after in-hospital cardiopulmonary arrest. *Resuscitation*, *133*, 47–52.

Kirkpatrick, D. L. (1976). Evaluation of training. In R. L. Craig (Ed.) *Training and Development Handbook, A Guide to Human Resources Development* (pp. 18.11–18.27). New York: McGraw-Hill.

Kirkpatrick, D. L. (1998). *Evaluating Training Programs*. San Fancisco: Berrett-Koehler.

Kirkpatrick, J. D., & Kirkpatrick, W. K. (2016). *Kirkpatrick's Four Levels of Training Evaluation*. Alexandria: ATD Press.

Krathwohl, D. R. (2002). A revision of Bloom's taxonomy, an overview. *Theory into Practice*, *41*(4), 212–218.

Lenguerrand, E., Winter, C., Siassakos, D., MacLennan, G., Innes, K., Lynch, P., … McCormack, K. (2020). Effect of hands-on interprofessional simulation training for local emergencies in Scotland, the THISTLE stepped-wedge design randomised controlled trial. *BMJ Quality & Safety*, *29*(2), 122–134.

Lydon, S., McDermott, B. R., Ryan, E., O'Connor, P., Dempsey, S., Walsh, C., Byrne, D. (2019). Can simulation-based education and precision teaching improve paediatric trainees' behavioural fluency in performing lumbar puncture? A pilot study. *BMC Medical Education*, *19*(1), 138.

Miller, C., Deckers, C., Jones, M., Wells-Beede, E., McGee, E. (2021). Healthcare simulation standards of best practice outcomes and objectives. *Clinical Simulation in Nursing, 58*, 40–44.

Molenda, M. (2003). In search of the elusive ADDIE model. *Performance Improvement, 42*(5), 34–37.

Molenda, M., Reigeluth, C. M., Nelson, L. M. (2003). Instructional design. In L. Nadel (Ed.), *Encyclopedia of Cognitive Science* (pp. 574–578). London: Nature Publishing Group.

Moreau, K. A. (2017). Has the new Kirkpatrick generation built a better hammer for our evaluation toolbox? *Medical Teacher, 39*(9), 999–1001.

O'Connor, P., Byrne, D., O'Dea, A., McVeigh, T. P., Kerin, M. J. (2013). "Excuse me," teaching interns to speak up. *The Joint Commission Journal on Quality and Patient Safety, 39*(9), 426–431.

O'Connor, P., Ryan, S., Keogh, I. (2012). A comparison of the teamwork attitudes and knowledge of Irish surgeons and US Naval aviators. *The Surgeon, 10*(5), 278–282.

Philips, J. J. (2003). *Return on Investment in Training and Performance Improvement Programs*. Oxford, UK: Butterworth-Heinemann.

Price, D. W., Wagner, D. P., Krane, N. K., Rougas, S. C., Lowitt, N. R., Offodile, R. S., … Lypson, M. (2015). What are the implications of implementation science for medical education? *Medical Education Online, 20*(1), 27003.

Prideaux, D. (2000). The emperor's new clothes, from objectives to outcomes. *Medical Education, 34*(3), 168–169.

Reid-McDermott, B., O'Connor, P., Carey, C., … Byrne, D. (2022). *A Compendium of the Steps Required to Complete 13 Essential Procedural Skills*. The Irish Centre for Applied Patient Safety and Simulation. Galway, Ireland: University of Galway.

Rudolph, J. W., Simon, R., Raemer, D. B., Eppich, W. J. (2008). Debriefing as formative assessment, closing performance gaps in medical education. *Academic Emergency Medicine, 15*(11), 1010–1016.

Thellen, U., Fraser, L., Jones, P., Leonard, P., Simpson, D. (2017). Regular in-situ simulation training of paediatric Medical Emergency Team leads to sustained improvements in hospital response to deteriorating patients, improved outcomes in intensive care and financial savings. *Resuscitation, 115*, 61–67.

Yardley, S., Dornan, T. (2012). Kirkpatrick's levels and education 'evidence'. *Medical Education, 46*(1), 97–106.

4 Scenario Writing

KEY POINTS

- The simulation scenario is a cornerstone of simulation-based education (SBE).
- Scenario writing occurs during the design phase of instructional design.
- Input on writing a scenario should be sought from a number of subject matter experts, from different healthcare specialities. In addition, input from patients and simulated participants (SP) may be sought.
- Take measures to avoid unconscious bias when writing scenarios.
- A structured approach should be taken to writing simulated scenarios.
- The first draft of a simulation scenario is very unlikely to be the final version of the scenario. A practice run, and regular updates are also required.

INTRODUCTION

The goal of simulation based education (SBE) is the creation of an authentic learning experience. The simulation scenario is a cornerstone of SBE. The scenario is generally an artificial representation of a real clinical event that has been modified to support learning. SBE has been described as 'theatre with a purpose' (Dieckmann et al., 2007). Using this analogy, the written scenario is the script for this theatre. Effective scenario design is crucial for team-based simulation, as well as simulations that use simulation participants (SPs) who represent patients, relatives or healthcare workers. Scenarios are generally not required for procedural or task-based simulations. Rather, this type of simulation requires a task analysis that outlines the specific steps required to perform the procedure. Guidance on conducting a task analysis is provided in Chapter 2.

CHAPTER OUTLINE

This chapter will provide guidance on scenario writing. Specific frameworks will be used to outline how to write scenarios for team SBE activities and for simulated participant (SP) SBE activities.

SCENARIO WRITING

Scenario writing occurs during the design phase of instructional design. Consistent with the model of instructional design outlined in Chapter 3, prior to writing a scenario, a training needs assessment should have been conducted, the learning outcomes/objectives identified, and that a simulation utilising a scenario is required in order to meet these outcomes/objectives. These activities, as well as others associated with instructional design, are discussed in detail in Chapter 3. There are also other considerations when designing a simulation scenario that are discussed later in the book – to include physical safety (Chapter 5), psychological safety and prebriefing (Chapter 6), and debriefing (Chapter 7).

A written scenario is a detailed description of a clinical encounter or event and is used to guide those running the simulation (faculty and technical staff), and ensure that the scenario aligns with the learning objectives of the SBE activity. An analogy that may be useful for scenario writing is to liken it to a recipe. The written scenario should include all of the ingredients for conducting the

DOI: 10.1201/9781003296942-4

simulation activity (e.g., learners, equipment), and also how they should be combined (e.g., the order in which activities should occur). Just as with a good cake recipe, it is important that the details of how things are to be done are provided in a scenario if it is to run without issue. The scenario should be written at a level of detail that someone who was not involved in developing the scenario is able to deliver the simulation session as envisaged by the authors of the scenario.

It is important to consider who should be involved in writing a scenario. Ideally, input should be sought from a number of subject matter experts from different healthcare specialities, to ensure that the scenario is factually correct and is an authentic representation of a real clinical event. Involving patients in writing scenarios, particularly in Simulated Participant (SP) scenarios, is becoming increasingly common. This involvement ensures that the patient voice is represented in the scenario (Chianáin et al., 2021). For example, we designed SP scenarios as part of a module on LGBTQ+ healthcare, which was developed for medical students. We engaged with members of the LGBTQ+ community in order to identify some of their challenges in accessing healthcare. We used this engagement to develop scenarios in which a medical student conducted a consultation with an SP playing a member of this community (e.g., the SP requests a prescription for Pre Exposure Prophylaxis; *PrEP*). Drawing upon the lived experience of members of the LGBTQ+ community allowed us to develop authentic, and relevant, scenarios (O'Connor & Byrne, 2022).

It is also important to try and avoid unconscious bias when writing scenarios. Unconscious, or implicit bias refers to ways people unknowingly draw upon assumptions about individuals and groups (Allen & Garg, 2016). We recently reviewed our scenarios with unconscious bias in mind and identified a number of issues. To illustrate, we found that the majority of our patients had traditional Irish names (e.g., Micheál, Kathleen,) and lacked diversity in their background. As a result, we have diversified the names/backgrounds of the patients in our scenarios and make greater use of our recently purchased dark skin tone manikins in our teaching. Another unexpected unconscious bias that was identified was how particular healthcare workers were portrayed. For example, the radiographer on-call would generally be unhelpful to the learners, and the surgeon would often be unable to review the patient when called by the learner (O'Connor & Byrne, 2022).

WRITING TEAM SIMULATION SCENARIOS

At the Irish Centre for Applied Patient Safety and Simulation (ICAPSS) we use a specific template for writing team scenarios. A blank version of this template is shown in Appendix 1. Below we will describe what should be addressed in the sections, and sub-sections, of this template when writing the scenario. The scenario is for the benefit of faculty and staff to ensure that everyone is 'on the same page' in terms of the purposed, objectives and progression of the scenario.

TITLE

The title should provide a clear explanation of the scenario. For example, "The management of post-op sepsis."

CASE SUMMARY

The purpose of this first section is to provide an overview of the scenario. This section has five headings:

- *Speciality* – identify the healthcare speciality, or specialties, for which the scenario is relevant (e.g., paediatrics, endocrinology, respiratory).
- *Target audience* – identify the target audience/learners (e.g., interns, recently graduated nurses, interprofessional learners).

- *Purpose* – provide an overall aim of the scenario. For example, *"the main target of the session is for learners to understand the roles of every person in the healthcare team in the management of an elderly patient with sepsis.* Other purposes might be *"to identify…, to escalate… etc."*
- *Keywords* – list some keywords for the scenario (e.g., *sepsis, elderly, post-op*).
- *Learning objectives* – the learning objectives for the simulation activity are listed. For example, *"apply the sepsis protocol"* (see Chapter 3 for a detailed discussion on writing learning objectives).

SCENE INFORMATION

This section provides some broad background to the scenario, and consists of four headings:

- *Location* – Identify the setting for the simulation (e.g., ward, emergency department) and whether it is to be carried out at simulation facility or in situ.
- *Participants per scenario* – Identify how many learners will participate in the scenario (e.g., two interns).
- *Duration of scenario* – State the expected duration of the scenario.
- *Duration of the debriefing* – State the expected duration of the debriefing.

FACULTY INFORMATION

This section provides a 'plot summary' for faculty, facilitators, and others who are responsible for running the scenario. This section should highlight any points of importance in the scenario (e.g., the patient's presentation and history, how the scenarios will progress, the expected actions of the learners). For example:

This scenario begins with a patient who is day 2 post-op removal of a tumour in his colon. The patient is starting to display signs of sepsis including shivering. His vital signs indicate a clinical deterioration. He also has a developing pneumonia which causes coughing and shortness of breath. When the interns enter, they should receive a handover from the nurse embedded participant who explains that the patient is feeling unwell today, 'like he has the flu' and that his early warning score has triggered a call to review him. The interns should examine the patient and take a brief history. Possible sites for this infection are a central line which will appear inflamed, the developing pneumonia and possibly post-op sepsis. The patient has a temperature spike, is breathing fast, has a high heart rate and low blood pressure. As the scenario develops, the patient will become more unwell. He becomes more confused. The intern learners should commence the sepsis 'give 3, take 3' protocol. Blood results will then be available which will confirm an infection. The interns should call the surgical/medical registrar and microbiology (or use the hospital guidelines) for advice on appropriate antibiotics. The scenario should end as the sepsis protocol has been completed and the interns have called for senior help.

INITIAL PATIENT INFORMATION

This section provides the initial information on the patient at the beginning of the scenario.

Patient Name:		Age:	Gender:	Weight:
Presenting Complaint:				
RR:	02 Sat: Fi02:	HR:	BP:	Temp:
Point of Care Glucose:		GCS:	Cap Refill Time:	EWS Score:
Triage note:				
Allergies:				
Past Medical History:		Current Medications:		

Additionally, this section should also contain a short description (generally read out by a facilitator) to orientate the learner to the simulated environment. This section should address who the learner is expected to be in the scenario, what day and time it is, who the patient is, what they have presented with, what investigations have already been completed, and what is expected of the learner or the task they are required to undertake. For example:

> You are the surgical intern. It is 2 p.m. on a Monday and you are being called to the ward to see John Williams, a 58-year-old male who is day 2 post removal of a large tumour in his colon. He is currently receiving intravenous fluids at 100 mL per hour and has complained to the nursing staff of feeling unwell and 'flu-like' since this morning. His Early Warning Score (EWS) is 6. All necessary notes are at the patients' bedside and nursing staff will be available to assist you if needed. You are to review the patient, conduct a focused history and examination and then formulate a differential diagnosis for the patient's complaints. You are to manage the situation as it develops.

FURTHER PATIENT INFORMATION

This section elaborates on the information included in the initial patient information section described above. It includes any potentially relevant information that was not included in the previous section that would be contained in the patient's medical records. For example, past medical and surgical history, medications and allergies, social history. This section should give key points and lines to the person voicing the manikin in the scenario and should aim to include answers to any questions the learners may ask. For example:

> Your name is John Williams, a 58-year-old male who has just had surgery 2 days ago to remove a tumour in part of your bowel. Today you have begun to feel 'hot and cold' with a cough and shortness of breath developing. You are anxious as it has been difficult for the last few days. You are upset as you thought you were recovering well post-op but now feel unwell and like this might be a setback. You feel 'like you have the flu'. You don't have any chest pain; you are not coughing up anything. You have no pain in your abdomen, noting that the nurse changed your wound dressing earlier and it looked 'in good shape'. The consultant said you can get the nasogastric tube taken out later and you are passing small amounts of wind. The nurse tells you that you have a temperature and that she is calling the doctor. When the doctor arrives, you can tell your history in full but are to remain anxious. You should cough occasionally and state that you 'feel hot and cold'. Eventually you become drowsier and more disoriented as the scenario progresses. You do not know where you are. You become more confused at the end of the scenario.

SUPPORTING TEAM OR FACULTY

This section is to provide information to the simulation team or anyone who is an embedded participant. In the section information is provided on:

- *Embedded participants* – the role(s) of any embedded participants should be identified (e.g., paramedic, nurse, receptionist). An embedded participant (EP) is an individual who is trained or scripted to play a role in a simulation encounter (Lioce et al., 2020). They also generally have a role in guiding the scenario to make sure it is progressing, and prevent it from deviating from the plan. For example, the EP may prompt a struggling learner to call for help, or they may address any unexpected problems (e.g., electrical plug becoming detached). Often an EP will have a radio and ear piece that allows them to receive communications instructions from the control room.
- *Technicians* – the number of technicians required to set up/teardown the scenarios and reset the scenarios.

This section also includes a script for the EP to hand over to the learner when they enter the scenario, i.e., what the embedded nurse/paramedic/family member will actually say to the learner. For example:

Hello Doctor. This is Mr. Williams, a 58-year-old male who was admitted for surgical removal of an obstructing tumour in his descending colon. He is now day 2 post-op. He was doing fine clinically until today when he began complaining of feeling unwell and flu-like. His EWS is 6. I have noticed he appears to be shivering in his bed quite a lot. He has a central line in situ and a stoma bag which is draining normally. He also has a urinary catheter which now has 40 mL of concentrated urine in it. His observation sheet is here and I have recorded the parameters and I noticed that he has a high temperature of 39 degrees C and increased work of breathing. All of his notes are at the bedside table. Can you please review him?

This section also includes prompts for anyone answering the phone who is part of the simulation team or faculty, if a call for help is initiated by a learner. This section includes a synopsis of what the person receiving the call should say. For example, if the call is to the blood bank then the EP answering the phone would ask for "Name, board/hospital number, Date Of Birth, How much blood do you need?" They might also ask "Have you sent a group and hold/cross match, do you require any other blood products etc?" If the incoming call is being made to other areas or disciplines, e.g., radiology, surgery, medicine etc., consideration needs to be given as to whether they would take this call and assist or direct elsewhere, what they would ask about this patient, or whether they would be available to come and help if asked. It is important that these issues are thought out ahead of time to ensure that, as much as possible, the response has been planned.

TECHNICAL/ENVIRONMENTAL REQUIREMENTS

This section is focused on the environment or situation where the scenario is located and the realism of the simulation. This section contains eight subsections which are discussed below.

- *Patient* – identify whether the patient is a manikin, simulated participant, or whether both are used (e.g., manikin and actor playing a family member). Any demographics or specifications should also be delineated (e.g., child). A manikin is generally used for team-based simulation. However, for some scenarios a simulated participant may be preferable. Scenarios that are focused on communication like psychiatry scenarios or scenarios that require examination of the neurological or musculoskeletal system may be better with an actor or simulated participant playing the part of a patient.
- *Patient appearance and set up* – describe (in detail) how the manikin is supposed to look for the technician setting up the scenario. For example, clothing, appearance, body position, whether they have peripheral lines inserted, a catheter, and/or dressings.
- *Special equipment* – identify any special equipment that is required for the scenario (e.g., spinal board and c-spine collar, arrest trolley). Larger pieces of clinical equipment such as defibrillators and infusion pumps should be the same as those the learners use in clinical practice so that they are not disorientated or confused by the equipment. A short overview as to their use should be part of the prebrief orientation. Consumables should also be the same as those used by the learners in clinical practice.
- *Medications* – any medications required for the scenario should be listed.
- *Moulage* – describe any moulage required for the patient. Moulage can improve realism for learners. For example, the application of moulage to simulate an open fracture in trauma scenarios or redness around a line to suggest cellulitis or a specific rash pattern in paediatric scenarios can support desired learning outcomes.
- *Paperwork and results* – laboratory, point of care and radiological results and images may be required for the learners to make decisions during the scenario. For example, the lactate on a venous or arterial blood gas may be useful in the management of a sepsis case. These pieces of documentation and paperwork can be generated using templates and given to the learners in paper format. Displaying these on a large screen for observing learners to see

helps them to remain engaged while watching the scenario. If using real clinical images or results, they must be de-identified. It is important that copies of these documents are included and stored with the written scenario.

- *Monitors at case onset* – indicate whether the patient is on a monitor with vitals displayed and the beginning of the case or not.
- *Patient reaction and examination findings* – include any relevant physical exam findings that require manikin programming or cues from patient. (e.g., abnormal breath sounds, sweating etc.).

SCENARIO STATES, LEARNER ACTIONS AND TRIGGERS

This section is concerned with describing the progression of the simulation scenario and what needs to happen in order for the scenario to move onto the next 'scene' or state. In the ICAPSS template (see Appendix 1) this is depicted as a table which addresses:

- Baseline vitals (e.g., respiratory rate, oxygen saturation, heart rate, blood pressure, temperature).
- Affect/behaviours (e.g., in distress, alert, agitated).
- Clinical signs (e.g., bilateral wheeze, no pulse in right foot, murmur).
- Expected learner actions (e.g., examination, history, request ABG/laboratory blood tests). Learner actions that lead to a response (triggers; e.g., when fluids are administered, then the BP will increase to X).

Each state is represented as a row in the table. It allows the faculty and technical staff to know when changes are required to the vitals, patient behaviour, and clinical signs and what these changes should be. Another important consideration is to include activities that provide insights into what the learning is thinking. These insights can be achieved through handovers, or phone calls to other healthcare providers. There may be only one or two states in some scenarios, or there may be multiple states in more complex scenarios where the patient is deteriorating rapidly. In the initial draft, there can be a tendency to try and put too much into a scenario. Particularly for junior learners, very little may need to actually happen in a scenario to achieve the intended learning objectives.

FURTHER CONSIDERATIONS FOR WRITING TEAM SCENARIOS

The first draft of a simulation scenario is very unlikely to be the final version of the scenario. Once a first draft is written, it should be circulated to other simulationists and subject matter experts for comment from both a practical and authenticity perspective. Once this input has been incorporated, it is also very important to do a practice run of the scenario to ensure that it can be completed as envisaged by the authors. The practice run will also lead to changes to the scenario, and it may be that more than one practice run is required. To some extent, a scenario is a 'living document'. Additions and changes may continue to be made based on the experience of running the scenario with learners. Adaptions will also be required if there are changes made to clinical practice. In addition to the scenario itself, and any required paperwork, additional information and guidance should also be included in the document. For example, written guidance on running the prebrief (see Chapter 6) or, debrief (see Chapter 7), or a picture of the manikin with the required moulage.

WRITING SIMULATED PARTICIPANT SCENARIOS

Many of the principles, and considerations, for writing a SP scenario are similar to those required to write a team simulation scenario. However, there is also one important difference. SP encounters general focus on the communication between the patient (SP) and the healthcare provider (learner).

Therefore, the SP needs to be provided with a sufficient 'back story' in order to be authentic as a patient and allow them to answer any of the learners' questions. The SP may need direction in how to respond or react to the learner (e.g., sad, angry) and they are also responsible for moving the scenario on to ensure that all of the learning objectives are met. SP encounters may also contain a specific post-encounter task that the learner has to perform after the initial communication encounter. These range from carrying out a clinical examination to performing a procedure or task (e.g., taking blood or writing a prescription) to handing over to another colleague or speaking to a relative. Having all of the information available for each of these parts is an important consideration for the author(s) of the scenario.

At the Irish Centre for Applied Patient Safety and Simulation (ICAPSS) we use a template for standardised participant scenarios; this template was developed by the Association of SP Educators (ASPE). A blank version of the template that we use is in Appendix 2; the latest version of the ASPE case development template is available from: www.aspeducators.org/aspe-case-development-template. There are multiple sections; not all are required for all SP scenarios and they can be deleted as required. The first three parts of the SP scenario template are discussed below as they are the main components required to create a scenario for a SP encounter.

OVERVIEW AND ADMINISTRATIVE DETAILS

The purpose of the first section is to provide a broad overview of the scenario for the SP, and ensure that the faculty running the scenario know how long it will take, and have any additional equipment that may be required. The subheadings that need to be completed in this section are outlined below.

• Patient/SP name	• Lay summary of patient story
• Name of the case/encounter	• Learning objectives
• Expectations of the learner	• Assessment instruments (e.g., rating checklist)
• Patient's reason for visit	• Event format and duration
• Patient's chief complaint	• Patient demographics
• Differential diagnosis	• Special supplies (e.g., medical device)
• Actual diagnosis	• SP reference materials (e.g., websites with information on the patient's condition)
• Case purpose or goal	
• Learner and discipline	• Special instructions for support staff
• Learner prerequisite knowledge and skills	

NOTES AND LEARNER INSTRUCTIONS

The next section of the scenario outlines the information the learner should receive before they commence the encounter. This is generally provided on a single sheet of paper for them to read which may be handed to them or may be on the door of the SP room. It may describe some/all of the elements below:

• Setting (including place and time)	• Patient's chief complaint
• Patient's name	• Vital signs (if applicable)
• Patient's age	• Laboratory results (if applicable)
• Patient's gender	• Image results (if applicable)

For example,

the patient you are about to meet is Mr. Simon Smyth, a 33-year-old male.

Today, Simon presents complaining of symptoms including fatigue, excessive urination and thirst. Blood glucose on fingerprick testing is 16 and urine dipstick is positive for glucose.

Simon previously attended your GP surgery five months ago for a check-up and was seen by a colleague in the practice. He has a family history of diabetes and high cholesterol. At that visit one of your medical colleagues saw Simon and requested fasting bloods and told Simon to make a follow-up appointment to review his blood results in two weeks. Simon did not make the follow-up appointment. Today, before you go in to see him, you review his blood results from 5 months ago and notice his fasting glucose was 10. There is nothing in the patient record to suggest that the patient was contacted to explain the abnormal blood test.

The learner should also be provided with some brief guidance on what they are expected to do during the encounter. For example: "*your role today is to: (1) greet the patient; (2) explain the findings and implications of the abnormal blood test; and (3) develop a plan for the future management of his condition*".

CASE CONTENT FOR SPs

This section provides detail on the 'patient's medical history and perspective' for the SP. It is likely to be quite detailed because, as described earlier, the SP has to be prepared to answer questions from the learner, react appropriately, and ensure that the encounter progresses as planned. Guidance should be provided on family history (e.g., relevant disease history in the family), social history (e.g., occupation, exercise, diet), any relevant physical exam findings. An example of a family history description is:

your mother and father are both living in London. Your mother has had diabetes for the last 15 years. You think she was diagnosed at age 45 and is on insulin and she has some problems with her eyes and kidneys. She attends a diabetes clinic regularly. You father has high cholesterol and is on medication. You have one brother who is healthy and married living in Australia. You moved to Galway when you were 20 years old.

This section also should include a detailed description of the demeanour of the patient, or any other special instructions. This should address:

- what the patient wishes to achieve from the visit. "*The purpose of this visit is to find out what is wrong with you, and find out when you will be well enough to return to work. Find out why you were not informed about the abnormal blood tests from five months ago, and receive an apology for this error on behalf of the practice from the doctor seeing you today.*"
- guidance on the patient's affect (e.g., sad, irritated). "*You are short and confrontational at the beginning of the interview and occasionally interrupt the doctor to voice your frustration.*"
- an initial opening statement and questions the patient must ask. "*So, I had diabetes 5 months ago, why didn't anyone call me?*"
- questions the patient will ask if provided the opportunity. "*If asked in an open-ended way why you are here, state: I'm feeling really awful and I never found out what my blood tests showed, could we have avoided all of this?*"

It is becoming increasingly common for the SPs to provide feedback to the learners in addition to, or sometimes instead of, a member of faculty. The ability of SPs to give immediate and specific feedback to a learner is one of the main advantages of using SPs as compared with real patients; SP feedback has been well received by learners (Qureshi & Zehra, 2020). If such feedback is to be used, just as is the case for assessors (see Chapter 8), the SP should be trained to provide feedback. It is also important to ensure that the focus should be on providing feedback from the patient's perspective – as this is the real uniqueness and strength of SP feedback (Bokken et al., 2009). Time should be spent practicing the delivery of feedback so that it is constructive, not too harsh and focuses on the patient's perspective. In addition, some guidance should be provided in the written scenario. For example, "*Consider how the learner informed you about the delayed diagnosis. Was this done in an empathetic way? Did you believe the learner was genuinely sorry?*"

FURTHER CONSIDERATIONS FOR WRITING SP SCENARIOS

At a minimum, the written draft of the scenario must be reviewed by a subject matter expert (to ensure the scenario makes sense from the perspective of the healthcare provider), an experienced SP (to ensure that there is sufficient information to allow someone to be the patient), and a patient (to ensure the patient is realistic and to avoid any stereotyping or unconscious bias). As with the team scenario, it is very important that at least one practice run of the scenario is completed before it is used with learners, with a focus on how to give feedback to learners if that is required. Consideration should also be given to whether written guidance should also be provided for how to conduct a debriefing (see Chapter 7). Further, as SP scenarios are often used for formal and/or summative assessment such as an Objective Structured Clinical Examination (OSCE), it is important that if a checklist or global rating system is to be used that it is included with the scenario. Assessment is discussed in detail in Chapter 8.

CONCLUSION

A well-written scenario is imperative for effective simulation-based education. A good scenario is not easy to write, and will take a number of drafts. It is also not something that should be done alone, and the development of an authentic and realistic scenario will require input from a range of stakeholders. Many simulationists will also be happy to share scenarios so that you can adapt them rather than starting from scratch. Given the work required to develop a scenario, we strongly recommend using a template and sharing scenarios with others.

FURTHER READING

Appendix 1 ICAPSS Team scenario development template.
Appendix 2. ICAPSS SP case development template.
Alinier, G. (2011). Developing high-fidelity health care simulation scenarios: A guide for educators and professionals. *Simulation & Gaming, 42*(1), 9–26.
O'Connor, P., Byrne, D. (2022). Diversity in healthcare simulation. *International Journal of Healthcare Simulation.* DOI: 10.54531/rgus8506.

REFERENCES

Allen, B.J., Garg, K. (2016). Diversity matters in academic radiology: acknowledging and addressing unconscious bias. *Journal of the American College of Radiology, 13*(12), 1426–1432.
Bokken, L., Linssen, T., Scherpbier, A., Van Der Vleuten, C., Rethans, J. J. (2009). Feedback by simulated patients in undergraduate medical education: a systematic review of the literature. *Medical Education, 43*(3), 202–210.
Chianáin, L. N., Fallis, R., Johnston, J., McNaughton, N., Gormely, G. (2021). Nothing about me without me: a scoping review of how illness experiences inform simulated participants' encounters in health profession education. *BMJ Simulation & Technology Enhanced Learning, 7*(6): 611–616.
Dieckmann, P., Gaba, D., Rall, M. (2007). Deepening the theoretical foundations of patient simulation as social practice. *Simulation in Healthcare, 2*(3), 183–193.
Lioce, L., Lopreiato, J., Downing, D., Chang, T.P., Robertson, J.M., Anderson, M., Diaz, D.A., and Spain, A.E., & the Terminology and Concepts Working Group. (Ed.) (2020). *Healthcare Simulation Dictionary.* Rockville, MD: Agency for Healthcare Research and Quality. Available from: https://www.ssih.org/Dictionary
O'Connor, P., Byrne, D. (2022). Diversity in healthcare simulation. *International Journal of Healthcare Simulation.* DOI: 10.54531/rgus8506
Qureshi, A. A., Zehra, T. (2020). Simulated patient's feedback to improve communication skills of clerkship students. *BMC Medical Education, 20*, 1–10.

5 Physical Safety in Simulation

KEY POINTS

- There is the potential of simulation to result in physical harm to patients, learners, simulated participants, and simulation facility staff in a range of unanticipated ways.
- The physical risks of healthcare simulation activities have received less attention than the psychological risks.
- In situ simulation is associated with a unique set of risks. Of particular importance are the risks to patients from medications and equipment that may not be intended for use in real patient care.
- Guidance for the identification and management of some physical risks can be found in the literature and through simulation societies. However, these must be unified into a comprehensive approach to manage health and safety, within the local context.
- Simulation facility staff should complete health and safety training courses that are relevant to their role such as manual handling, first aid, fire safety etc.

INTRODUCTION

There is a potential for simulation activities to result in physical harm to patients, learners, simulated participants, or simulation facility staff. Risks can emerge in unanticipated ways and as such can be hard to predict. These potential risks should be addressed in the health and safety policy for the facility, and as part of the planning process for a simulation activity.

Within the simulation literature, the majority of the focus is on the psychological safety of learners and participants. This is discussed in detail in the next chapter. Here we address issues related to physical safety within simulation. This is an important but often-overlooked aspect of simulation practice/activity. It is worth noting that a safe work environment is one of the key domains in the Association of Standardized Patient Educators (ASPE) Standards of Best Practice (Lewis et al., 2017).

CHAPTER OUTLINE

This chapter will:

- identify the potential physical risks to patients, learners, simulated participants, and facility staff; and
- describe the development of a simulation facility safety policy.

PHYSICAL SAFETY OF SIMULATION

It is vital that simulation activities are conducted in a manner that minimises the risk of physical harm to the users and staff of a simulation facility. To this end, there are important health and safety issues that must be considered before, during, and after a simulated activity. Moreover, different

DOI: 10.1201/9781003296942-5

safety issues and risks will be of concern depending on whether the simulation activity is occurring in a designated simulation facility or in the real clinical environment. Either way, it is important that simulationists develop a safety policy to proactively identify, and mitigate, the physical safety risks associated with simulation activities.

RISKS TO PATIENTS

The term in situ simulation is used to describe simulation that takes place in a real clinical environment. This type of simulation poses specific risks to patients that must be considered. If the simulation activity is being carried out in a 'working' unit such as a ward, or the Emergency Department (ED), there is the potential for interference with the clinical care being delivered to patients. This poses the questions: Is it appropriate to conduct simulation training in the clinical environment at all? and, At what point do the risks outweigh the benefits of in situ simulation? To answer these questions, it is worth briefly considering the purpose and efficacy of in situ simulation.

IN SITU SIMULATION – PURPOSE AND EFFICACY

In situ simulation is the practice of carrying out simulation activities in the actual clinical environment. In situ simulation offers an opportunity to evaluate, assess, and train in the environment where the work is done. As such, in situ simulation is a very effective approach for testing system processes and identifying latent safety threats that may be hidden in the care system (see Chapter 11 for a discussion). In situ simulation is also useful for practicing teamwork and communication with a native clinical team within the context of the real clinical setting.

While evidence of the efficacy of in situ simulation is still emerging, existing research is promising and suggests that the blending of learning in the work environment can have positive impacts on team process and organisational learning outcomes (Rosen et al., 2012). The benefits of this type of simulation are particularly important in high-acuity situations that demand the coordination of many healthcare providers, healthcare systems and resources. Until recently, research reporting the direct impact of in situ simulation on patient outcomes has been scarce but recent systematic review studies have demonstrated a significant improvement in morbidity and/or mortality outcomes following integrated in situ simulation training (Goldstein et al., 2020). "In-situ simulation has the potential to improve reliability and safety in high-risk clinical areas by allowing participants to practice and reinforce skills in their own working environment, during their scheduled work hours" (Bajaj et al., 2018: 221). However, although in situ simulation has the potential to improve patient safety, there are also risks to carrying out simulation in an active clinical space that must be managed.

RISK OF INTERFERENCE WITH REAL PATIENT CARE

Healthcare departments are always busy and, by their nature, high acuity units will benefit from in situ simulations designed to test the system (Bajaj et al., 2018). However, in situ simulation activities such as unannounced mock codes (i.e., a simulated cardiac arrest in a hospital) have the potential to disrupt patient care, by taking staff and resources from the care of real patients (see Example 5.1).

In situ simulation has the advantage of being on site, so staff do not have to take time to travel to a dedicated off-site simulation facility. Nonetheless, in situ simulation is time-consuming and those running in situ simulations must be sensitive to working conditions on the unit so that decisions can be made about whether to run a simulation session or not. A go/no-go decision should be based on clear criteria. Bajaj et al. (2018) offer key essentials for the development of "no-go considerations" for planned in situ simulation.

EXAMPLE 5.1   EXAMPLE OF DISRUPTION TO PATIENT CARE RESULTING FROM IN SITU SIMULATION

Active shooter simulation. A simulated active shooter drill was planned for a military medical centre. However, when the alert was sent out there was no indication that this was a simulation event. Therefore, a real response was trigged to include a full police reaction, lockdown of the medical centre, and evacuation of patients. No-one was physically injured, but the event was frightening for the people involved.

(adapted from Foundation for Healthcare Simulation Safety, FHSS; healthcaresimulationsafety.org/incidents/)

- *Staffing needs*: The clinical unit should be adequately staffed for that shift, taking into consideration staff-to-patient ratios and patient acuity.
- *Workflow patterns*: In situ simulations should not be held during shift changes, sign outs, or during scheduled procedures, nor should it require staff who are involved in high-risk patient procedures or care at the time of the simulation.
- *Clinical load/acuity*: Consideration should be given to both the volume of patients as well as the acuity and complexity of patients and any scheduled procedures.
- *Equipment needs*. In situ simulations should not use equipment that is low in stock in the unit.
- *Unanticipated events*: In order to protect the psychological safety of staff, in situ simulations should be postponed if a serious clinical event occurs in the unit on the same shift as the planned simulation.

The interprofessional nature of in situ simulations requires that these "no-go" considerations be made for all disciplines and departments that are involved in the simulation activity. Along with the considerations themselves, the process of making these decisions is also important. The process should be collaborative, transparent, clearly communicated to all staff, and should be reviewed and updated periodically.

RISK ASSOCIATED WITH THE USE OF MEDICATION

Simulation scenarios often involve the use of medication. There are three options for using medication in simulation:

1. use real in-date medications;
2. use fake medication (e.g., saline or water); or
3. use manufactured simulated medications that closely resemble real medications but do not contain an active drug (e.g., tablets, ampoules, inhalers).

Each of these three options comes with their own risks and these should be carefully considered when designing simulation-based education (SBE). The main risk is the use of medications in simulation. This is particularly true for simulation activities conducted in the real clinical envirnment where this is a risk of 'contamination'. Contamination occurs when fake, or simulated, medications are inadvertently administered to an actual patient. This can happen in any number of ways and it may be difficult to predict the potential pathways of contamination (see Example 5.2).

EXAMPLE 5.2   INTRODUCTION OF SIMULATED INTRA-VENOUS (IV) FLUID INTO THE CLINICAL ENVIRONMENT (ROBYN ET AL., 2015)

In 2014, a number of clinical facilities in the US inadvertently ordered simulated intra-venous (IV) fluid, instead of real IV fluid from a manufacturer. The simulated IV fluid bag closely resembled a real IV fluid bag. The real IV bag was labelled with "PRACTI-0.9% Sodium Chloride" while the simulated version was labelled with "Practi-Products for Clinical Simulation". In both cases, the labels were printed in letters less than 2 mm in height under the company logo. No additional warnings or markings on the simulated IV fluid bag indicated that it should not be administered to patients. A total of 45 patients erroneously received the simulated fluid, including two patients at an urgent care facility. Although neither patient died, both patients required hospital treatments, and one developed sepsis (Robyn et al., 2015).

The consequences of contamination are potentially serious for patients. In addition, there is the potential for medical negligence claims and/or reputational damage for the simulation programme. Torrie et al. (2016) suggest several strategies for controlling contamination.

- Manage all medications (simulated, fake or real) as required for real medications. Engage with pharmacy staff to ensure that procedures align with clinical practice. This includes the correct disposal of medications.
- Keep real medications in a locked cupboard or storage area.
- Create separate systems for the purchasing, handling, and storage of simulated and fake medicines, with tracking of supplies and disposal (similar to systems for managing hazardous substances).
- Use warning labels and stickers to highlight that the drug is for 'simulation use only'.
- Develop systems for pre-reconciliation and post-reconciliation of all medications used in a simulation. A formal pre- and post-simulation 'count' is an appropriate (but not infallible; see Example 5.3) approach to preventing inadvertent contamination of the real clinical environment or the transport of medications used in simulation back to a clinical area. Additionally, requiring learners and staff to empty their pockets on departure will be particularly important if learners do not change clothes before returning to clinical areas.

Torrie et al. (2016) concluded that only real medications should be used during in situ simulation. "Given the risk of contamination, we recommend that real medications are always used for in-situ simulation. This opinion has been strongly supported by pharmacy staff in our institution" (Torrie et al., 2016: 919). However, some hospital pharmacy departments will only supply medications for patient use and not for education and training. Also, it may be that the real drugs are very expensive, or in short supply. So, there may be ethical considerations with using particular medications or real products for the purposes of simulation. However, what is most important is that a proper risk

EXAMPLE 5.3   ACCIDENTAL INJECTION WITH REAL ADRENALINE AUTOINJECTOR

As part of a primary school class on allergies and emergency response, pupils were given training in the use of adrenaline auto-injectors. A real auto-injector had become mixed in with the training devices. As a result, an 11-year-old boy administered himself with a dose of adrenaline. He was treated in hospital, and thankfully made a full recovery.

(adapted from FHSS; healthcaresimulationsafety.org/incidents/)

assessment is carried out prior to the simulation activity, and procedures are in place to mitigate the likelihood of fake or simulated drugs inadvertently getting into the real clinical environment.

The practice of using real but time-expired medications has also been described in the literature (Torrie et al., 2016). This is sometimes done for the purpose of reducing costs. However, this is not a recommended practice. Firstly, learners must be asked to ignore the expiry date during simulation which may reinforce bad practice. Secondly, expired drugs may pose even more risk to patients than fake or simulated drugs and for this reason we do not support this practice.

RISKS ASSOCIATED WITH THE USE OF SIMULATED AND REAL MEDICAL DEVICES AND MEDICAL EQUIPMENT

The use of real and simulated clinical equipment also poses a potential risk. For example, defibrillator cables designed for use on manikins could end up on a crash cart intended for real patient use. Similar to medication use discussed above, there are three options for the use of medical devices and equipment in simulation:

1. use real medical devices and clinical equipment that is serviced and certified for use with real patients;
2. use decommissioned real medical devices and equipment, which is not serviced and does not have a current certification for use with real patients; or
3. use simulated medical devices or equipment (e.g., a breathing circuit with mask and tracheal tube, pulse oximetry probe, carbon dioxide sample line and oxygen hose) which are not designed for real patient use.

Ensuring that clinical equipment, whether it is for simulation use only or safe for use with patients in the clinical setting, is labelled correctly and clearly, is vital for the safety of staff, learners, and patients (see Example 5.3). The departments responsible for the maintenance of clinical equipment in hospitals (e.g., Medical Physics, Clinical Engineering) should be consulted about the safe use and maintenance of clinical equipment in a simulation facility. Any large pieces of medical equipment (e.g., ventilators) that are real and also for use with patients, need to be included on a hospital record and service list and should be located in a single, accessible place so that they can be easily retrieved by hospital staff if required for patient use. Such equipment must be plugged in at all times so that it is fully charged should it be needed urgently. The same considerations given to the risk associated with the use of drugs in simulation should also be applied to medical devices and equipment.

RISKS ASSOCIATED WITH PATIENT RECORDS

Care needs to be taken with ensuring that fake patient records do not erroneously get into the hospital system (see Example 5.4). For written notes, every page should be clearly labelled 'for simulation

---

EXAMPLE 5.4   SIMULATED PATIENT ENTERED INTO A MEDICAL RECORD SYSTEM

An administrator mistakenly entered the demographics details of a manikin 'patient' into the hospital electronic medical record system. The error was caused by poor communication between administration and those responsible for the training. It took 18 hours of work to remove the fictitious manikin patient.

(adapted from FHSS; healthcaresimulationsafety.org/incidents/)

use only'. Also, if any real patient imaging or data is used (e.g., ECGs, X-rays) then care must be taken to ensure that any identifiable information is removed.

RISK OF INAPPROPRIATE USE OF HOSPITAL RESOURCES

There is a risk that real hospital systems and processes can be activated during simulations to the detriment of real patient care. Phone calls activating real emergency teams can happen in highly immersive simulations. To illustrate, there are many examples of resuscitation teams, blood banks, or first responders being mistakenly called during a simulation activity (Raemer et al., 2018). In other cases, clinical personnel may not have responded as quickly to a call believing – erroneously – that it was part of a simulation event and so a rapid response was not required. This 'cry wolf' phenomenon is a risk when mock codes are run in an organisation. As an example, one of the authors was involved in a situation in which a military diver displayed the symptoms of an arterial gas embolism (AGE) following a dive. This is a relatively uncommon event, but is simulated fairly frequently to ensure that the dive team is able to respond appropriately. In this case, the team assumed that this was just another simulation, so their reaction to the diver was not as rapid as it would have been if the team had known the diver was experiencing a real AGE. Fortunately, the delay was not too great, the diver was treated, and he made a full recovery. Overall, care needs to be taken not to cause a "cry wolf" reaction in the healthcare setting. Phone lines in a simulation facility should be disconnected from the hospital phone system and clearly labelled with the number to use. In the case of mock codes, the switchboard as well as management should be made aware that the mock code is being conducted. Finally, consideration must be given to the pros and cons of announcing, or not announcing, a simulated event such as a mock code to the participants.

RISK OF NEGATIVE TRANSFER

Another more subtle risk to patients associated with simulation is that of "negative transfer". We know that simulation is a powerful tool for learning and that knowledge, skills, and behaviours learned in simulation translate to clinical practice. Negative transfer describes the amplification of poor practice during a simulation which then transfers out into clinical practice. Negative transfer can occur when short cuts are taken during a simulation to improve efficiency, which are then transferred to the clinical setting. For example, reusing certain pieces of equipment/consumables during a simulation to save money may mean that the learner does not get to experience how challenging it is to open the packaging while maintaining good infection control practices. This practice may also leave the impression that reusing the item is appropriate. Other examples of negative transfer include not insisting that learners wear gloves for certain procedures, not checking the expiry date on drugs or Personal Protective Equipment (PPE), or inadvertently suggesting to learners that such practices are unnecessary. The incorrect or inadequate stocking of emergency carts and trollies in a simulation facility can confuse learners as well as suggest that cart accuracy and consistency is unimportant. Similarly, a poor medication choice made in a simulation scenario that is not addressed during a debriefing might leave a learner with the impression that the choice was appropriate (Raemer et al., 2018).

RISKS TO LEARNERS

It is important to consider the physical risk to learners from participating in a simulation. These risks are generally no greater than those in the clinical environment (e.g. use of live equipment, sharps, and medications). However, these risks should be considered as the learner may be less vigilant during an education or training session than they would be in the clinical setting, or they may assume that all equipment in a simulation facility is 'not real'. It is important that the learners do not become complacent to these clinical risks just because they are in a simulated setting. To illustrate, in our simulation centre we use real defibrillators that are charged and fully functional; therefore, there is a risk of shocking a learner if appropriate controls are not in place. These risks arc particularly relevant to junior learners who may be more at risk of harm (e.g. needlestick injury) as they may be still learning the task. While every effort should be made to ensure that the clinical equipment in a simulation facility is the same as is used in clinical practice, that is not always possible and some of the equipment may be unfamiliar to the learners. Extra vigilance, demonstration of equipment use during the prebriefing, and clear labelling of equipment are all required to ensure that the learners do not receive an injury.

RISKS TO SIMULATED PARTICIPANTS

The risks to Simulated Participants (SP) largely arise when they are playing the part of a patient within a scenario, during which it is possible that an over-exuberant learner could cause physical harm to them. This is particularly true if there is a requirement for a physical examination of the SP. An example might be repetitively manipulating the joints of an old or frail simulated participant, eliciting reflexes and neurological signs multiple times in patients, or any kind of internal exam (e.g. examining the ear canal) of an SP. These risks may need particular consideration in an Objective Structured Clinical Examination (OSCE) exam during which a relatively large number of junior learners may repeat the same exam on a SP and moreover they may perform the task poorly – resulting in the potential for injury. Clear written instructions to the learner, sufficient SPs, and adequate breaks during OSCEs to allow SPs to rest are important ways to avoid fatigue and injury.

RISKS TO SIMULATION FACILITY STAFF

The simulation facility staff have the potential for physical injury from moving and lifting heavy equipment and from slips, trips, and falls. For example, manikins can weigh up to 100 kg. Therefore, it is important that centre staff receive manual handling skills training, and that lifting equipment is available if required (e.g. patient hoists). Importantly, large equipment should not be stored at a height. Staff may also handle potentially hazardous biological and chemical agents such as bleach, dyes, cadaveric material, or animal parts. Therefore, it is important that the risks associated with these substances and materials are known and managed. As with the other risks outlined in this chapter, it is important that a simulation facility has appropriate risk management processes in place in order to identify and manage these risks. Some of these processes can be adapted from those in use in hospitals, for other risks, processes in use in laboratories may be more appropriate. All staff should have fire safety and first aid training so they are trained and prepared to respond if required. There are online chemical management systems (e.g., www.safedoc.ie/) that can be used by simulation facility staff to access safety information on the chemical products used in their facility. Safety data sheets and other risk assessment tools are available on these systems in order to assess and manage chemical risks.

DEVELOPING A SIMULATION FACILITY SAFETY POLICY

Simulation facilities must develop a comprehensive set of policies and procedures and mechanisms to protect the physical and psychological safety of all individuals involved in simulation. In addition, organisations must have an effective policy management system which outlines a consistent approach to policy development, review, approval, and documenting. Brazil et al. (2022) describe the process they used to develop the simulation safety policy at their institution. A first step is to consider whether a single or separate policies are required for "centre-based" or in situ simulation activity. They opted for a single policy, with detailed content focused on in situ simulation issues.

However, in other circumstances separate policies may be warranted. Based upon their experience, Brazil et al. (2022) provide useful recommendations for developing the safety policy for a simulation facility. We expand on these recommendations with our experience below.

FORM A STEERING GROUP FOR DEVELOPMENT AND IMPLEMENTATION OF THE SIMULATION SAFETY POLICY

It is important that a broad range of stakeholders are involved in the development of the safety policy. This should include input from facility staff, faculty, and other users of the facility. It is also important to solicit guidance from a pharmacist and medical physics/medical engineering to ensure any associated risks with drugs or medical devices are adequately addressed.

IDENTIFY EXISTING SAFETY PROCEDURES FOR THE HEALTH SERVICE/EDUCATIONAL INSTITUTION THAT ARE RELEVANT FOR THE SIMULATION FACILITY

It is generally not necessary to develop a completely new set of safety policies and procedures for a simulation facility. Many simulation facilities are part of a larger parent organisation that will already have safety policies and procedures in place to address many identified risks. To illustrate, the Irish Centre for Applied Patient Safety and Simulation (ICAPSS) is a simulation facility that serves both the University of Galway and Galway University Hospital. From a safety management perspective, ICAPSS is under the jurisdiction of the University of Galway Health and Safety Management System. The university has formal structures which address many generic health and safety issues associated with running laboratories (e.g. chemical handling). Therefore, the relevant university policies are referenced as part of the ICAPSS policy. For other risks the Galway University Hospital policy may be more appropriate (e.g. for the disposal of sharps and medical waste or the handling of medications). Where it is necessary to develop completely new procedures, these should be designed in a way that is consistent with those from the parent organisation (Brazil et al., 2022).

INCORPORATE EXISTING SIMULATION SAFETY PRACTICES

Brazil et al. (2022) recommend adapting generic resources to meet the needs of a specific simulation facility. As outlined earlier, this may be by adapting the policies or procedures from the parent organisation of the simulation facility. Additionally, simulation societies such as the Society for Simulation in Healthcare (SSH) and FHSS provide resources and guidance covering various risks but these need to be unified into a comprehensive approach to manage health and safety, within the local context. For example, Dongilli et al. (2021) have developed a useful simulation programme policy and procedures manual template that identifies 23 different areas that may need to be addressed- one of which relates to safety and security (see Chapter 9 for a discussion). Brazil et al. (2022) also recommend incorporating the "pledge" of best practices for simulation programmes to reduce simulation related hazards from the FHSS (see Table 5.1).

CONSIDER THE HAZARDS AND EXTENT OF PREDICTED SAFETY RISK BASED ON THE LITERATURE AND LOCAL EXPERIENCE

The literature may be useful in identifying risks that you may not have considered. However, there will still be local context and local activities which may create unexpected or unanticipated risks. For example, the ICAPSS is situated at the rear of a hospital. On a rare hot day in Ireland, a confused patient wandered out of his ward in the hospital and into the simulation centre and was unexpectedly found in one of the teaching rooms. This situation had occurred because the doors (which normally require swipe-card access) had been propped open to aid airflow.

TABLE 5.1
FHSS 'Pledge' of Best Practices

1. Label all medication, supplies, and equipment to indicate whether they are for human use or not.
2. Educate all faculty and staff about potential hazards resulting from simulation exercises.
3. Inform participants about potential hazards to patients, participants, and staff.
4. Periodically review simulation programmes and scenarios and facilities for potential threats to safety and initiate mechanisms to mitigate them.
5. Vet teaching to make sure that short cuts are not legitimised through simulation such as not wearing gloves.
6. Vet teaching to ensure that incorrect information is not left unchecked in the debriefing discussion.
7. Educate those who conduct simulations outside of the facility about simulation safety issues.
8. Have rigorous process for returning equipment or supplies back into the clinical environment in a safe and appropriate way.
9. Maintain an open and transparent reporting system for simulation safety violations and near-misses and accidents.
10. Give priority to simulation safety over cost, expedience, and fidelity in decision-making.

Source: healthcaresimulationsafety.org/

PRIORITISE MEDICATION SAFETY AND LIAISE WITH PHARMACY REPRESENTATIVES

As discussed earlier in this chapter, there is the potential for harm from medications used in simulation activities. Therefore, it is important that pharmacists are consulted in developing medication safety procedures. We would also suggest extending this recommendation to consulting medical physics/engineering on medical device safety.

EFFECTIVELY COMMUNICATE THE EXISTENCE OF THE SIMULATION SAFETY POLICY, AND THE NEED FOR STAFF INVOLVED IN SIMULATION DELIVERY TO COMPLY

There is little point in having a policy if the facility staff are unaware of it. Therefore, it is important that the staff are aware of the policy, know how to access it, and are familiar with the content. A single location for policies and procedures, training records, and risk assessments is desirable. It is also important that an induction programme for new staff should include content on health and safety, a list of mandatory staff training requirements, and should also be included in any annual staff training. The policies and procedures must also be reflective of "work as done" rather than "work as imagined". That is, the policies and procedures must be practical and support staff to work safely, rather than an idealistic approach to safety management that cannot be practically applied.

ENABLE SIMULATION FACULTY TO CONDUCT SAFE SIMULATION SESSIONS THAT ARE COMPLIANT WITH THE POLICY

Leading on from the previous point, it is important that staff and faculty are compliant with the policy, and there is a culture at the facility of following the policy. Again, this is more likely to be achieved if the policy is consistent with "work as done".

DEVELOP A REPORTING PROCESS FOR SIMULATION-RELATED ADVERSE EVENTS OR NEAR-MISSES, PREFERABLY INTEGRATED WITHIN THE HEALTH SERVICES' CLINICAL ADVERSE EVENT REPORTING FRAMEWORK

It is important that any adverse events and near-misses are reported, rigorously investigated, and any issues identified addressed. Generally, the larger organisation of which most simulation facilities are a part will already have processes in place for reporting and investigating near-misses and adverse events.

CONCLUSION

There is the potential for simulation activities to result in physical harm to patients, learners, simulated participants, and centre staff. These are risks that should be identified, and mitigated or managed, and every facility should have a health and safety folder that contains their safety policy, staff health, and safety training records and a health and safety induction presentation that is an overview of the activities, for new staff members.

In situ simulation, in particular, may have specific, and potentially serious, risks to patients. It is also important to consider that if serious harm was to occur at a simulation facility, this could have reputational implications for the simulation community more broadly. Therefore, it is very important that, in addition to the psychological risks, we also consider the physical risks of healthcare simulation.

FURTHER READING

Bajaj, K., Minors, A., Walker, K., Meguerdichian, M., Patterson, M. (2018). 'No-go considerations' for in-situ simulation safety. *Simulation in Healthcare*, *13*(3), 221–224.

Brazil, V., Scott, C., Matulich, J., Shanahan, B. (2022). Developing a simulation safety policy for translational simulation programs in healthcare. *Advances in Simulation*, *7*(1), 1–7.

Lewis, K.L., Bohnert, C.A., Gammon, W.L., Hölzer, H., Lyman, L., Smith, C., Thompson, T.M., Wallace, A., Gliva-McConvey, G. (2017). The association of standardized patient educators (ASPE) standards of best practice (SOBP). *Advances in Simulation*, *2*(1), 1–8.

Raemer, D., Hannenberg, A., Mullen, A. (2018). Simulation safety first: an imperative. *Advances in Simulation*, *3*(1), 1–4.

ONLINE RESOURCES

- Foundation for Healthcare Simulation Safety (FHSS) for information and best-practice strategies to mitigate the risks associated with simulation in healthcare: http://healthcaresimulation safety.org.

REFERENCES

Bajaj, K., Minors, A., Walker, K., Meguerdichian, M., Patterson, M. (2018). "No-go considerations" for in-situ simulation safety. *Simulation in Healthcare*, *13*(3), 221–224.

Brazil, V., Scott, C., Matulich, J., Shanahan, B. (2022). Developing a simulation safety policy for translational simulation programs in healthcare. *Advances in Simulation*, *7*(1), 1–7.

Dongilli, T., Gavilanes, J., Shekhter, I., Kuki, A., Wong, J., Howard, V., Hara, K., Lin, M. (2021). *SSH Simulation Program Policy and Procedure Manual Model Template*. Minneapolis, MN: Society for Simulation in Healthcare.

Goldstein, D., Krensky, C., Doshi, S., Perelman, V. S. (2020). In-situ simulation and its effects on patient outcomes: a systematic review. *BMJ Simulation & Technology Enhanced Learning*, *6*(1), 3.

Lewis, K. L., Bohnert, C. A., Gammon, W. L., Hölzer, H., Lyman, L., Smith, C., Thompson, T. M., Wallace, A., Gliva-McConvey, G. (2017). The association of standardized patient educators (ASPE) standards of best practice (SOBP). *Advances in Simulation*, *2*(1), 1–8.

Raemer, D., Hannenberg, A., Mullen, A. (2018). Simulation safety first: an imperative. *Advances in Simulation*, *3*(1), 1–4.

Robyn, M. P., Hunter, J. C., Burns, A., Newman, A. P., White, J., Clement, E. J., … Blog, D. (2015). Adverse events associated with administration of simulation intravenous fluids to patients - United States, 2014. *Morbidity and Mortality Weekly Report*, *64*(8), 226.

Rosen, M. A., Hunt, E. A., Pronovost, P. J., Federowicz, M. A., Weaver, S. J. (2012). In-situ simulation in continuing education for the health care professions: a systematic review. *Journal of Continuing Education in the Health Professions*, *32*(4), 243–254.

Torrie, J., Cumin, D., Sheridan, J., Merry, A. F. (2016). Fake and expired medications in simulation-based education: an underappreciated risk to patient safety. *BMJ Quality & Safety*, *25*(12), 917–920.

6 Psychological Safety and Prebriefing

KEY POINTS

- Unsurprisingly, SBE can provoke anxiety in learners. This anxiety can interfere with learner engagement.
- Careful consideration should be given to the creation of a safe learning environment.
- Psychological safety should be considered for everyone involved in a simulation-based education activity – regardless of their role.
- Although psychological safety should be considered at every stage of a simulation-based education activity, the prebriefing is a particularly important stage in the creation of a safe learning environment.

INTRODUCTION

There is a large body of research demonstrating that participating in simulation-based education (SBE) can cause high levels of stress and anxiety for learners. To illustrate, Emergency Medicine (EM) residents participating in a simulation of a critically ill patient scenario were found to have a mean increase in heart rate of 42 beats per minute, and a mean systolic blood pressure increase of 23 mmHg during the simulation as compared to baseline assessment (Kharasch et al., 2011). Other studies have found that simulation participants report high levels of self-reported stress and anxiety (Müller et al., 2009), and significant elevations in stress markers such as salivary α-amylase and cortisol (Müller et al., 2009; Pottier et al., 2011). These findings are unsurprising; learners are aware that their performance is being watched by their peers and they are conscious that there will be an analysis of their performance afterwards in the debrief. Thus, learners may feel that there is a risk to participation in SBE. This feeling of mental threat that arises out of participation in SBE has been defined as 'psychological risk' by Rudolph et al. (2014). High levels of stress may have negative consequences on learner performance, and the learning experience (Al-Ghareeb et al., 2017). As such, careful consideration should be given to creating a learning environment that learners perceive to be psychologically safe.

CHAPTER OUTLINE

In this chapter we describe the concept of psychological safety, identify threats to psychological safety in SBE, outline the notion of a safe learning environment, and suggest how this can be established during the prebriefing for a SBE activity.

PSYCHOLOGICAL SAFETY

Psychological safety is a perquisite to learning in SBE (Rudolph et al., 2006). Psychological safety can be defined as a feeling (explicit or implicit) within the context of a simulation-based activity that participants are comfortable participating, speaking up, sharing thoughts, and asking for help as

DOI: 10.1201/9781003296942-6

needed without concern for retribution or embarrassment (Lioce et al., 2020). Another useful definition of psychological safety is: the perception of members of the team that the team is safe for risk taking, and mistakes will be considered learning opportunities rather than causing embarrassment or punitive consequences (Edmondson, 1999; Higgins et al., 2012). However, SBE has some unique characteristics that threaten the psychological safety of learners. These threats are detailed below.

THREAT TO PROFESSIONAL IDENTIFY

SBE may require learners to engage in a learning activity in which they are not completely proficient. Moreover, the learners in the simulation activity are aware that their performance may be critiqued in the debriefing. It is understandable, then, that professional learners who value their professional identity may worry about performing poorly in front of their peers or that their performance will be seen to fall below an acceptable standard. This perceived threat to professional identify can undermine learner engagement with simulation and risks undermining the educational value of the session. For this reason, Rudolph et al. (2014) state that "reducing threats to professional and social identity is increasingly recognised as the sine qua non of learning in groups" (p. 340).

THREAT OF VALIDITY

A simulation mimics the real clinical environment. However, every aspect of the simulation will not be exactly the same as the real world. Some learners may find the 'pretend' aspect of simulation problematic, with some people more willing to 'buy in' than others. Learners that do not buy in, or who find the realism of the simulation problematic, can become defensive about their performance and may blame deficits in performance on the realism of the simulation, resulting in an undermining of the educational value of the SBE activity.

THREAT OF HIDDEN AGENDAS

Learners may worry that *they will be tricked or misled* as part of SBE. This can lead them to behave in a way that differs from their normal practice. For example, they may be reluctant to make decisions or take action as they believe these will be 'used against them' in the debriefing. The learners may also spend time searching for the 'hidden agenda' and this may interfere with the progress of the simulation event and the learning opportunity.

THREATS ASSOCIATED WITH PARTICULAR TYPES OF SCENARIOS

Maintaining psychological safety is important in all SBE activities. However, there are three particular types of scenarios for which we recommend extra caution. These are: (i) scenarios which utilise deception, (ii) scenarios in which there is a planned (or unplanned) death of the simulator, and (iii) scenarios with a focus on equality, diversity, and inclusion.

SCENARIOS THAT UTILISE DECEPTION

There are many different forms of deception. A common scenario is for a learner to be given an incorrect drug or drug dosage, or where a simulated healthcare practitioner in the simulation deliberately acts inappropriately. The onus is on the learner to identify the error or poor behaviour and 'speak up'. This kind of deception is a high-risk strategy for educators to use because if the learner fails to act this may damage their self-image and lead to self-recrimination or defensiveness in the debrief. Therefore, it is important that if deception is used, it should be carefully considered and managed.

Proponents of use of deception argue that a certain amount of deception is inherent in simulation and that deception is sometimes necessary to generate a genuine psychological experience that the learner can then apply to real clinical practice. Another argument is that deception can be used to generate a "healthy scepticism among learners about the perfection of fellow clinicians" (Calhoun et al., 2015: 165). Opponents to deception argue that it can erode the trust between educators and learners which is essential to effective SBE. Moreover, deception amplifies the power differential between educator and learner and its use negates any consent or agreement that was established between educator and learner (Calhoun et al., 2015).

We are not opposed to the use of deception, and recognise that it may be necessary to achieve certain learning objectives (e.g., encourage the checking of drug dosages). However, we recommend great care when using deception in SBE and advise that if deception is part of a simulation it is made clear to the learners during the prebrief. Overall, the use of deception in simulation should be:

- used in a considered way and in the context of a well-developed and thought-out scenario;
- used with experienced facilitators;
- used when there is no other way to achieve the learning outcomes;
- used in such a way that avoids learners feeling that they have been unnecessarily 'tricked' and treated unfairly;
- discussed in the prebriefing to alert the learners; and
- justified in the debriefing to explain why the deception was necessary in order to achieve the learning outcomes.

Overall, the onus is on the simulationist to manage these potentially problematic aspects to simulation and to create a learning environment that is 'psychologically safe' in which learners are willing to take risks and open themselves up to critique. Extra time may be required in the debriefing to address the use of deception and to ensure that the learners understand why it was necessary and do not feel they have been tricked or unfairly treated. The goal is not to create an environment that lacks challenge but to create an environment where learners are tested but not threatened, so that the educational benefit is maximised.

DEATH OF THE SIMULATOR SCENARIOS

Another potential contentious issue for SBE is simulator death. Approaches can vary from never allowing the simulator to die unless death is the objective of the scenario, to allowing the simulator to die unexpectedly during any scenario. Corvetto and Taekman (2013) have identified three different types of simulated death:

1. *Death is expected by the facilitator and the learner* – managing a death is a learning outcome of the scenario, and there is awareness by all that the patient will die (e.g., end-of-life care scenario);
2. *death is expected by the facilitator and unexpected by the learner* – managing a death is a learning outcome of the scenario, but not expected by the learner (e.g., unanticipated respiratory complications); and
3. *death is unexpected by the facilitator and the learner* – death results from the action or inaction on the part of the learner (e.g., failing to manage anaphylaxis episode appropriately).

Similar to deception, our recommendation is that if death is part of a simulation event, it should be done with care, forethought, and by skilled facilitators. Corvetto and Taekman (2013) have a number of recommendations for how to incorporate simulator death into SBE:

- ensure the readiness of the facilitator to debrief a scenario that includes the death of the simulator – individual facilitators may differ in their level of comfort in debriefing;
- take particular care in planning the prebriefing for a death scenario – the fact that death is a possibility should be made clear;

- do not allow simulator death with early-stage learners – as early-stage learners are unlikely to have experienced death in the clinical setting, it is not recommended that they experience it in the simulator;
- allow simulator death only with advanced learners;
- do not use simulator death as punishment for poor performance – if managing a death is not a learning outcome, but the learners' actions or inactions would result in the death of the patient in real life, then the simulation activity should be stopped early, and addressed in the debriefing;
- balance the emotions of the learners – the potential for emotional distress should be anticipated when using simulation to teach about death, it is recommended that a simulation facility should have a protocol in place for responding to a distressed learner;
- perform a careful debriefing – learners should be given the time and space to share their concerns, thoughts, and feelings and appropriately skilled facilitators should provide support as needed (Rudolph et al., 2007); and
- prioritise psychological safety over learning – it is important that psychological safety is considered in the planning, prebriefing, and debriefing.

Corvetto and Taekman (2013) provide additional recommendations for a simulated death that is unexpected by the learners and facilitators:

- follow a predefined protocol for an unexpected death – just as it is recommended that there is a protocol for responding to a distressed learner, a simulation facility should also have a protocol in place for managing an unexpected death; and
- make extra time during the debriefing – the unexpected death will likely require extra time to debrief to ensure that the learners understand what happened, and are given the opportunity to ask questions.

Equality, diversity, and inclusion (EDI) Scenarios

Healthcare simulation is increasingly being used to support EDI efforts in healthcare to address issues of access and quality of care faced by diverse communities. To illustrate, we developed some formative simulation sessions as part of a module on LGBTQ+ healthcare for medical students. We engaged with members of the LGBTQ+ community in order to identify some of their challenges in accessing healthcare. We used this information to develop scenarios in which a doctor conducted a consultation with a simulated participant playing a member of this community (the scenario involved a patient asking a General Practitioner for a prescription for Pre Exposure Prophylaxis; *PrEP*). Drawing upon the lived experience of members of the LGBTQ+ community allowed us to develop authentic, and relevant, scenarios (O'Connor & Byrne, 2023).

There is the potential for EDI-focused simulation scenarios to impact the psychological safety of the simulated participants (e.g., they may experience conscious or unconscious bias from the learners), the learners (e.g., they realise they have beliefs about other people that might not be right or reasonable), and the facilitator (e.g., they are uncomfortable about their ability to debrief EDI scenarios). The Sim-Edi tool (Purdy et al., 2021) provides useful guidance in supporting these types of reflections not just in EDI-focused simulations, but should EDI issues be raised in any SBE session.

Threat to the Psychological Safety of Simulated Participants

It is not only the psychological safety of the learners that requires consideration; in some SBE activities it is also necessary to consider the psychological safety of simulated participants (SPs). To illustrate, we ran a simulation in which an SP played the part of a pregnant mother who has been in a road traffic accident, and whose older child had been badly injured. The SP told us that this scenario had affected her for the rest of the day as she reflected upon the circumstances of the woman she had

TABLE 6.1
ASPE Safe Work Environment Principles and Practices

Safe work practice

- Ensure safe working conditions (e.g., number of rotations, breaks, psychological challenges of the role).
- Anticipate and recognise potential occupational hazards.
- Screen SPs to ensure they are appropriate for the role.
- Allow SPs to opt out of any activity if they feel it is not appropriate for them to participate.
- Ensure SPs are clear about the guidelines and parameters of a simulation activity.
- Provide SPs with strategies to mitigate potential adverse effects of role portrayal.

- Inform SPs about the criteria and process to terminating a simulation if they feel it is inappropriate or harmful.
- Structure time and create a process for de-roling and/or debriefing.
- Monitor for, and respond to, SPs who have experienced adverse effects of participation in an activity.
- Provide a process for SPs to report adverse effects.
- Support SPs who act in accordance with programme expectations if a complaint is made about them.
- Manage learner expectations of an SPs possibilities and limitations
- Clearly define the expected scope of SP involvement.

Confidentiality

- Understand the specific principles of confidentiality that apply to each simulation event.

- Ensure the SPs understand and maintain the principles of confidentiality related to the activity.
- Protect the personal information of all stakeholders.

Respect

- Respect SPs' self-identified boundaries (e.g., limits to physical touch).
- Provide SPs with adequate information so they can make informed decisions about participation.

- Ensure the SPs understand if and how they will be compensated.

Source: Adapted from Lewis et al., 2017.

been playing in the scenario. Moreover, SPs may be asked to play a role that is similar to a situation that they have experienced themselves (e.g., a cancer diagnosis), which they may find upsetting. In addition, SPs may be exposed to poor practice, insensitive interactions, learners who overstep the boundaries of the simulation.

The Association of Standardized Patient Educators (ASPE) identified standards of best practice for simulation that involves SPs (Lewis et al., 2017). These standards consist of five domains: (1) safe working environment; (2) case development; (3) SP training; (4) programme management; and (5) professional development. The safe work environment domain is particularly relevant to the psychological safety of simulated participants. The principles and practices in this domain are summarised in Table 6.1, and provide a useful overview of psychological safety considerations for SPs.

ESTABLISHING A SAFE LEARNING ENVIRONMENT

Lioce et al. (2020) define a safe learning environment as one of mutual respect, support, and respectful communication among leaders and learners; where open communication and mutual respect for thought and action are encouraged and practiced. It is an environment where learners feel physically and psychologically safe to make decisions, take actions, and interact in the simulation. Rudolph et al. (2014) adds to the concept of a safe learning environment with the concept of a 'safe container for learning'. This metaphor is used to imply a controlled and bounded space in which learners feel "secure enough to be uncomfortable or trust that they will have help managing difficult feelings and anxiety" (Rudolph et al. 2014: 340).

The metaphor of a 'safe container' has benefits in focusing educators on the construction of SBE activities in a way that protects the psychological safety of learners. Yet there are a number of caveats to the usefulness of this metaphor. First, the notion of the safe container is somewhat misleading as it implies that simulation is a 'closed system' were nothing must leak in or out. However, clearly the aim of SBE is for the learning to translate to the real clinical environment. Thus, there should be a desire for learned knowledge, skills, and behaviours to leak out of the learning container. Second, it should also be acknowledged that things also leak into SBE activities. Individuals and clinical teams bring their past experiences and team culture into the SBE activity. For example, if a strict hierarchy is observed within the team, this will likely emerge in the simulation activity. Similarly, if a culture of disrespect is normal in the clinical environment this will transfer to the simulation setting. Team culture can pose a challenge for the simulationists, but also represents an opportunity to identify and shed light on a negative culture that may lead to positive change.

Rudolph et al. (2014) suggest that creating a safe container for learning begins in the prebriefing for the SBE activity. While this is true from the learners' perspective, from the educators' perspective, much of the groundwork in establishing the safe learning environment begins even before this – in the planning and development stage – where educators consider the ethical and psychological aspects of the simulation, in advance (Gaba, 2013).

PREBRIEFING

Lioce et al. (2020) describe a prebriefing as:

> an information or orientation session held prior to the start of a simulation activity in which instructions or preparatory information is given to the participants. The purpose of the prebriefing is to set the stage for a scenario, and assist participants in achieving scenario objectives.
>
> *(p. 37)*

This is all certainly true. However, the prebriefing is also the stage in a SBE activity where a safe learning environment should be established for the learners. A scoping review found that a prebriefing resulted in: significant improvement in psychological safety and learner confidence; reductions in learner stress; improvements in skills and knowledge acquisition; and a more reflective and constructive debriefing (El Hussein et al., 2021).

There are two types of information to impart to learners in the prebrief: (i) describing what learners can expect in the SBE activity; and (ii) describing what is expected from learners in the session (Rudolph et al., 2014).

DESCRIBING WHAT THE LEARNERS CAN EXPECT DURING THE SBE ACTIVITY

If learners know what to expect it will lessen their anxiety and set the learner up to engage fully with the simulation.

Rules of Engagement

Learners need to know the rules of engagement in the SBE activity. This can be considered a learning contract or agreement between the learners and the educators whereby the learners agree to participate fully in the scenario and in the debriefing and the instructors agree to provide feedback with respect and genuine curiosity (Rudolph et al., 2008). Part of the rules of engagement should be to let learners know if performance evaluation is formative or summative (see Chapter 8). This will affect the learner's attitude towards the session and the perceived threat level in relation to their performance.

Facilitator Stance

Closely aligned to the rules of engagement is the stance taken by the facilitators. At the Centre for Medical Simulation in Boston, they call this stance the 'basic assumption' and it conveys a positive presumption about the abilities of the learners. The basic assumption they declare to their learners is: "we believe that everyone participating in this simulation is intelligent, capable, cares about doing their best, and wants to improve" (Rudolph et al., 2008). This is a powerful statement, as it sets the conditions for a full and frank debrief and will enhance learners' willingness to examine and discuss their actions critically and openly.

Clearly Stated Goals

The goals of the SBE activity should be clearly described to the learners. For some simulations, this does not necessarily mean that all of the learning objectives are communicated to the learners as this may compromise the learning from the activity. However, the learners should be provided with an overview of the activity and the goals of the session. For example, rather than telling the learners they will be expected to manage a patient with sepsis, they may be told that they will be managing an acutely unwell patient. The learners must also be made aware of whether the evaluation is a formative or summative assessment (see Chapter 8 for a discussion of assessment).

Confidentiality

Everyone who is present at the SBE activity should be identified by name and role and their interest in the session should be clarified to the learners. If an observer is present it should be made clear who they are and why they are observing. It may be that they are observing faculty and not learners and this should be clarified. Usually, it is made clear that performance in the simulation is treated confidentially. Therefore, the learners' performance will not be discussed outside of the SBE activity, and learners themselves should not discuss their own performance, or that of others, outside of the session. If video-recording will be used for the debriefing this should be conveyed to the learner. How these videos will be used and if they will be retained must be clear to the learners.

Properties and Functionality

Learners should have the opportunity to become familiar with the simulation environment (i.e., the simulation space they will be using), equipment, monitors, and the simulators that will be use in the SBE activity. Centre staff should clarify the properties of the simulators and their functionality. Mori (1970) coined the term 'uncanny valley' to describe a phenomenon where, as robots become more technologically advanced and increasingly human-like, there is a point at which they become close to human, but are not quite right. It is proposed that slight differences can be more distracting than if the robot was less human-like. It is suggested that familiarising the learners with the simulators and with larger pieces of equipment during the briefing may help to limit this effect. We have also found that we must show medical students how to use a landline telephone as they have never seen one before.

Process and Timings and Logistical Details

Logistical elements of the SBE activity may seem trivial to faculty and simulation facility staff, but can be a big distraction to learners if not clarified early in the session. Learners should know about coffee and lunch breaks, how long the session will last and each element of the session.

Describing What Is Expected of the Learners

In addition to outlining what learners should expect, there are also expectations of the learner that should be clarified. SBE is experiential learning which necessitates active participation and engagement in the activity. Therefore, SBE places some unique demands on the learner.

Fiction Contract

In order to get the most out of SBE, learners must be willing to enter into a 'fiction contract' with instructors whereby they agree to 'pretend' that this is a real clinical environment in order to fulfil the goals of the learning event. Learners must also agree to 'suspend their disbelief' and play a role and 'pretend' that the patient and situation is real so as to be able to immerse themselves in the simulation. Instructors agree to make the environment as realistic as possible and to be transparent and clear about the limitations to the realism. Some learners are more willing and able to enter into this contract than others, but experience suggests that the quality of the learning experience will depend on the learner's willingness to engage as fully as possible. One way to inspire learners to engage in the fictional contract is to remind learners that, although some aspects of the environment are not real, the case is or may be based on a real clinical case and one that they may encounter in the future.

Expectation to Participate and Engage

Usually, there is an expectation that all learners will participate in the scenarios. However, this will depend on the size of the learner group and whether the opportunity to participate is present. Mandatory simulation activities require that all learners get exposure and should be factored into resource planning where large numbers exist e.g., undergraduate medical students. The issue of volunteering should also be clarified. Will everyone be expected to participate in the simulation activity or will volunteers be sought? Instructors should have a clear strategy for dealing with unwilling participants. Instructors should also be clear that learners are expected to work within their own capabilities and scope of practice.

It is suggested that a simulation facility should have a standardised prebriefing that is used at the facility. To illustrate, the prebriefing that is used in Clinical Skills Centre at Great Ormond Street Hospital for Children covers five areas:

1. facilitator stance;
2. establishing a secure setting (e.g., ensuring all staff meet the learners, sharing the logistical plan, orientating learners to the simulation environment);
3. exploring simulation experiences (e.g., finding out if learners have had a negative experience of simulation in the past);
4. agreeing learning objectives (e.g., outline the course objectives, informing learners if they will be assessed); and
5. discussing the fictional contract.

Clearly, it will not always be necessary to go through each of the points described above in the prebriefing for every SBE activity. For example, an Emergency Department that runs regular weekly SBE will not need to address every point each time a session is run. Similarly, a SBE session focused on teaching suturing techniques using a skin pad simulator will also not require an extensive prebriefing. Therefore, some pragmatism and flexibility is required. The Debriefing Assessment for Simulation in Healthcare (DASH; Brett-Fleegler et al., 2012) tool discussed in Chapter 7 can also be used to provide feedback to a facilitator on their prebriefing.

CONCLUSIONS

Psychological safety is an important consideration for SBE. It needs to be considered in all phases of a SBE activity – planning and development, prebriefing, during the simulation, and in the debriefing. It also must be considered for everyone involved in a simulation – learners, simulated participants, faculty, and technical staff. It could be argued that as healthcare workers may experience upsetting events in their work, they should also be exposed to these scenarios in a simulated environment so that they are ready to meet these challenges when they experience them clinically. We do not disagree with this premise. However, SBE differs from the real world, and there is a responsibility to the learners to ensure that their psychological safety is protected in an educational environment.

FURTHER READING

Calhoun, A. W., Pian-Smith, M. C., Truog, R. D., Gaba, D. M., Meyer, E. C. (2015). Deception and simulation education: issues, concepts, and commentary. *Simulation in Healthcare, 10*(3), 163–169.

Rudolph, J. W., Raemer, D. B., Simon, R. (2014). Establishing a safe container for learning in simulation: the role of the presimulation briefing. *Simulation in Healthcare, 9*(6), 339–349.

ONLINE RESOURCES

• Purdy, E., Brazil, V., Symon, B. SIM-EDI: a tool for sim team reflexivity. 2021; Available from: https://icenetblog.royalcollege.ca/2021/09/14/equity-diversity-and-inclusion-in-simulation-a-reflexive-tool-for-simulation-delivery-teams/

REFERENCES

Al-Ghareeb, A. Z., Cooper, S. J., McKenna, L. G. (2017). Anxiety and clinical performance in simulated setting in undergraduate health professionals education: an integrative review. *Clinical Simulation in Nursing, 13*(10), 478–491.

Brett-Fleegler, M., Rudolph, J., Eppich, W., Monuteaux, M., Fleegler, E., Cheng, A., Simon, R. (2012). Debriefing assessment for simulation in healthcare: development and psychometric properties. *Simulation in Healthcare, 7*(5), 288–294.

Calhoun, A. W., Pian-Smith, M. C., Truog, R. D., Gaba, D. M., Meyer, E. C. (2015). Deception and simulation education. Issues, concepts, and commentary. *Simulation in Healthcare, 10*(3), 163–169.

Corvetto, M. A., Taekman, J. M. (2013). To die or not to die? A review of simulated death. *Simulation in Healthcare, 8*(1), 8–12.

Edmondson, A. C. (1999). Psychological safety and learning behavior in work teams. *Administrative Science Quarterly, 44*: 350–383.

El Hussein, M., Harvey, G., Kilfoil, L. (2021). Pre-brief in simulation-based experiences: a scoping review of the literature. *Clinical Simulation in Nursing, 61*: 86–95.

Gaba, D. M. (2013). Simulations that are challenging to the psyche of participants: how much should we worry and about what? *Simulation in Healthcare, 8*(1), 4–7.

Higgins, M, Ishimaru, A, Holcombe, R, Fowler, A. (2012). Examining organizational learning in schools: the role of psychological safety, experimentation, and leadership that reinforces learning. *Journal of Educational Change, 13*(1), 67–94.

Kharasch, M., Aitchison, P., Pettineo, C., Pettineo, L., Wang, E. E. (2011). Physiological stress responses of emergency medicine residents during an immersive medical simulation scenario. *Disease-a-Month, 57*(11), 700–705.

Lewis, K. L., Bohnert, C. A., Gammon, W. L., Hölzer, H., Lyman, L., Smith, C., ... Gliva-McConvey, G. (2017). The association of standardized patient educators (ASPE) standards of best practice (SOBP). *Advances in Simulation, 2*(1), 1–8.

Lioce, L., Lopreiato, J., Downing, D., Chang, T.P., Robertson, J.M., Anderson, M., Diaz, D.A., Spain, A.E., & the Terminology and Concepts Working Group. (Eds.) (2020). *Healthcare Simulation Dictionary (second edition)* (pp. 19–20). Rockville, MD: Agency for Healthcare Research and Quality. AHRQ Publication No.

Mori, M. (1970). The uncanny valley. *Energy, 7*(4), 33–35.

Müller, M. P., Hänsel, M., Fichtner, A., Hardt, F., Weber, S., Kirschbaum, C., ... Eich, C. (2009). Excellence in performance and stress reduction during two different full scale simulator training courses: a pilot study. *Resuscitation, 80*(8), 919–924.

O'Connor, P., Byrne, D. (2023). Fostering diversity in healthcare simulation. *International Journal of Healthcare Simulation.* DOI: 10.54531/rgus8506

Pottier, P., Hardouin, J. B., Dejoie, T., Bonnaud, A., Le Loupp, A. G., Planchon, B., LeBlanc, V. (2011). Stress responses in medical students in ambulatory and in-hospital patient consultations. *Medical Education, 45*(7), 678–687.

Purdy, E., Brazil, V., Symon, B. (2021). SIM-EDI: A Tool for Sim Team Reflexivity. Available from: https://icenetblog.royalcollege.ca/2021/09/14/equity-diversity-and-inclusion-in-simulation-a-reflexive-tool-for-simulation-delivery-teams/

Rudolph, J. W., Raemer, D. B., Simon, R. (2014). Establishing a safe container for learning in simulation: the role of the presimulation briefing. *Simulation in Healthcare*, *9*(6), 339–349.

Rudolph, J. W., Simon, R., Dufresne, R. L., Raemer, D. B. (2006). There's no such thing as "nonjudgmental" debriefing: a theory and method for debriefing with good judgment. *Simulation in Healthcare*, *1*(1), 49–55.

Rudolph, J. W., Simon, R., Raemer, D. B., Eppich, W. J. (2008). Debriefing as formative assessment: closing performance gaps in medical education. *Academic Emergency Medicine*, *15*(11), 1010–1016.

Rudolph, J. W., Simon, R., Rivard, P., Dufresne, R. L., Raemer, D. B. (2007). Debriefing with good judgment: combining rigorous feedback with genuine inquiry. *Anesthesiology Clinics*, *25*, 361–376.

7 Debriefing

KEY POINTS

- Debriefing is the most important element of simulation-based education (SBE).
- The mechanism of learning in debriefing is through reflection.
- Without debriefing to support the reflective process no real learning will occur.
- Debriefing provides a means for learners to traverse through the experiential learning cycle.
- Many models of debriefing exist, so the chosen approach should match the learning needs and the objectives of the session.
- Following a structured approach to debriefing ensures that all important phases of the debrief are achieved and will maximise the learning from the debrief.
- Choice of the conversational strategy to use in the analysis phase of the debrief is an important consideration as this will determine the substance of the analysis.
- The quality of the debrief is highly dependent on the skill of the facilitator. Thus, training and development of debriefing skills is important
- Peer coaching has the potential to transform every debrief into an opportunity for learning and development.

INTRODUCTION

It is clear from the previous chapters that considerable preparation, planning, and development goes into designing simulation scenarios and setting up the simulation event. Yet simulation without debriefing does not lead to learning; therefore, debriefing deserves as much preparation and planning as the rest of the simulation event (Motola et al., 2013). The purpose of debriefing is to support learners to reflect on their experiences in order to generate insights and learning that can be integrated into future performance. There is no one 'correct way' of conducting a debrief; however, there are a common set of key principles that should be observed in order to maximise the learning from the session (Rudolph et al., 2008).

CHAPTER OUTLINE

This chapter will:

- describe the purpose of debriefing and relate it to the phases of the experiential learning cycle;
- discuss the evidence-based strategies for effective debriefing;
- identify strategies for preventing and mitigating difficult debriefing situations;
- discuss the idea of debriefing as a formative assessment; and
- discuss approaches to developing debriefing skills.

DOI: 10.1201/9781003296942-7

WHAT IS DEBRIEFING?

Debriefing is a reflective discussion, or conversation, that occurs after a learning experience has occurred. During a debrief the experience is reviewed, areas for improvement are discussed and the learning from the experience is extrapolated to the real environment. Debriefing conversations may occur between learners and facilitators, or among the learners themselves, or some combination of both. Debriefing should be designed as an interactive, reflective conversation.

The importance placed on debriefing reflects the idea, originally proposed by Kolb (1984) in his experiential learning theory, that we do not learn from experience, we learn from reflecting on experience. Thus, without debriefing to support the reflective process, no real learning will occur. For this reason, debriefing is recognised as a necessary component of every simulation event (INACSL Standards Committee 2016; Motola et al., 2013). Motola et al. (2013) put it succinctly when they say: "without a post event reflective process, what the participants have learned is largely left to chance leading to a missed opportunity for further learning and making the simulation encounter less effective" (p. 1514). Debriefing is defined in the simulation dictionary as a formal, collaborative, reflective process within the simulation learning activity (Lioce et al., 2020).

REFLECTION

The mechanism of learning during debriefing is through reflection. Reflection involves looking back on events or experiences, analysing those experiences, extrapolating the learning from those experiences, and considering how this learning could be applied to future practice. Simulation-based education (SBE) is recognised as the ideal medium for developing reflective practice as it is a low-risk environment which can be managed, and learners can be coached through the reflective process (Schön, 2017). Reflective practice is recognised to have many benefits for professional development (Fanning & Gaba, 2007).

DEBRIEFING AND THE EXPERIENTIAL LEARNING CYCLE

It is helpful to consider debriefing in the context of the experiential learning cycle proposed by Kolb (1984) (see Chapter 2 for a detailed overview of experiential learning theory). The experiential learning cycle distinguishes four phases in the learning cycle: (1) concrete experience; (2) reflective observation; (3) abstract conceptualisation; and (4) active experimentation. In SBE, participation in the simulation scenario is the concrete experience. Participation in the debrief is the mechanism for learners to engage in reflective observation. The debrief also provides the opportunity for abstract conceptualisation when learners are encouraged to consider the relevance of the SBE experience to real clinical practice and identify where new insights can be incorporated into future action. Active experimentation can happen in the same simulation activity if learners have the opportunity to apply their learning in a new scenario or case, and ideally this will continue beyond the session into the real clinical environment. Thus, it can be seen that the debrief provides the venue for learners to traverse through the stages of the learning cycle (Fanning & Gaba, 2007).

PSYCHOLOGICAL SAFETY AND DEBRIEFING

Psychological safety was discussed in detail in Chapter 6, but it is worth reiterating that effective debriefing relies on the full engagement of the learners and this, in turn, relies on a safe, non-threatening and confidential learning environment. The foundation for establishing a psychologically safe learning environment should occur in the prebrief (see Chapter 6). However, it is recommended that at the beginning of the debrief the facilitators reiterating the 'basic assumption' that learners are competent and capable and trying to do their best; and also inform the learners about the structure, strategy, and approach that will be used in the debrief. The goal is to create a "supportive climate where students feel valued, respected, and free to learn in a dignified environment" (Fanning & Gaba, 2007).

DEBRIEFING STRATEGIES

A large amount of experience and knowledge has been amassed about how to optimise the learning from the debrief. For example, Sawyer et al. (2016), in their comprehensive analysis of debriefing strategies, identify several different factors that should be considered. Similarly, Ross (2021) identifies 12 evidence-based tips for effective simulation debriefing. Grant et al. (2018) present a toolbox for managing difficult debriefing situations. We have distilled the experience and knowledge into seven key strategies, and associated elements, that support effective debriefing. This information is summarised in Table 7.1, and discussed in more detail below.

STRATEGY 1: ADDRESS THE LEARNING OBJECTIVES

It is good educational practice to have clear learning outcomes and learning objectives for each simulation event. As discussed in Chapter 3, learning outcomes are broad in scope, and related to the entire SBE activity. In contrast, learning objectives are specific and detailed and relate to the specific knowledge, skills, and attitudes that should be covered in the debrief; they will provide the standard against which performance can be compared. Effective learning objectives will be specific, observable, achievable, appropriate, and easy to assess (Rudolph et al., 2008). Examples of effective objectives might be: "the team identifies and articulates roles and tasks for each team member", "the team takes a structured approach to patient management", "the team identifies and follows the

---

TABLE 7.1
Strategies for Effective Post-Simulation Debriefing

Debriefing Strategies	Elements
1. Address the learning objectives	• Good objectives are: specific, observable, achievable, appropriate and easy to assess
2. Structure the debriefing – use a structured framework	• Reactions • Description • Analysis • Summary
3. Select appropriate conversational techniques/ educational strategies	• Learner self-assessment • Facilitated discussions • Directive feedback • Blended approaches
4. Timing the debrief	• Within-event debriefing • Post-event debriefing
5. Utilise skilled facilitators	• Debriefing with good judgement • Manage time • Use open-ended questions • Use silence
6. Video-assisted debriefing	• Explain the purpose of viewing the clip • Provide examples of good practice • Use the clip as a launching pad for discussion
7. Standardised and scripted debriefing	• To support both the structure and the strategy of the debrief

correct procedure to ... ", or "the team articulates the diagnosis and the clinical priorities". It is not always necessary to share the learning objectives with the learners, if by doing so you would undermine what you hope to achieve in the session. Irrespective of whether the objectives are explicitly stated to the learners, they should always be addressed in the debrief. When debriefing is used as a formative assessment, objectives provide the standard against which performance is compared, and they allow for clear feedback when there is a discrepancy between actual and desired performance.

STRATEGY 2: STRUCTURE THE DEBRIEFING

Using a structure to guide the debriefing conversation has been shown to improve learning outcomes (Cheng et al., 2013). Several different debriefing structures exist, and they are well described in the literature. The choice of the best structure may depend on the purpose or objectives of the training and the skill or experience of the debriefers. Table 7.2 provides a brief overview of some of the more commonly used and well-described structures. Below we have used a four-phase approach to describing a debriefing structure in more detail: (1) reactions; (2) description; and (3) analysis; and (4) summary.

Reactions Phase

Recall how, in Chapter 6, we discussed how emotionally charged SBE can be for learners. The purpose of the reactions phase is to allow this emotion to be released so that a less emotionally charged debrief can occur. The facilitator will open the debrief with an open question such as 'How are you feeling?'. This will allow participants the opportunity to express or vent their emotions. In this initial phase it is good practice to allow all of those who were participants participated in the simulation the opportunity to express their emotions. Facilitators can then allay any worries or concerns raised by demonstrating respect for learners and by equating them to other similar groups of learners (Rudolph et al., 2008). Another benefit of the reactions phase is that it will highlight issues that are important to, or troubling for, learners. These issues should be noted and discussed in more detail later in the debrief.

Description Phase

During the description phase learners should be invited to summarise what happened during the simulated event. The facilitator may ask an open question such as "Can someone summarise the events in this case?" or "What was the medical issue in this case and what strategies were used to resolve it?" If the learners missed something important the facilitator can communicate this so that

---

TABLE 7.2
Commonly Used Debriefing Structures

Debriefing with Good Judgement Rudolph et al. (2006)	1. Reaction; 2. Analysis; and 3. Summary.
Gather, Analyse & Summarise (GAS model) Phrampus and O'Donnell (2013)	1. Gather; 2. Analyse; and 3. Summarise.
The Diamond Model Jaye et al. (2015)	1. Description; 2. Analysis; and 3. Application.

Promoting Excellence and Reflective Learning in Simulation
  (PEARLS)
  Eppich and Cheng (2015)
	1. Reaction; 2. Description; 3. Analysis; and 4. Summary.

Team-Guided. Self-Correction, Advocacy-Inquiry, and
  Systemic-Constructivist (TeamGAINS)
  Kolbe et al. (2013)
	1. Reactions; 2. Discuss clinical component; 3. Transfer from simulation to reality; 4. Discuss behavioural skills; 5. Summary; and 6. Supervised practice.

there is no confusion about what happened. The aim of this phase is to ensure that participants and faculty are in agreement and have a shared understanding of what happened during the simulated event. Similar to the reactions phase, facilitators should listen for issues that can be probed in greater detail in the next phase of the debrief.

Analysis Phase

During this phase the facilitator supports the learners to reflect on what happened during the simulated event in order to develop insights into why the learners acted the way they did. Learning occurs when facilitators and learners identify flawed or faulty mental models and work together to develop more appropriate practices or knowledge structures for the future. The analysis phase is supported by utilising an appropriate conversational technique or strategy to guide the discussion. The strategy chosen may depend on the experience level of the learners, the experience of the facilitator, and/or the objectives of the session. Conversational strategies are discussed in detail in the next section of this chapter.

Summary Phase

The summary phase of the debriefing is where the learning derived from the simulated event and the debrief are consolidated into learning points or take home messages that learners may apply in future practice. It may be conducted using a learner-centred approach such as "what learning will you take away from this case?" or in a facilitator-led approach where the educator provides an overview of the main take home messages: "the key learning points from this case were_____" However, using this approach, the educator is unable to determine if the learner's take-home messages align with the learning objectives of the session, and so the learner-guided approach is considered preferable. Another question to elicit take-home messages is "given another simulation like this, or a similar real situation, what would you do differently?" You may also have time to explore some barriers and enablers to the implementation of the learning into the work setting.

STRATEGY 3: SELECT AN APPROPRIATE CONVERSATIONAL STRATEGY

Several conversational strategies for debriefing are described in the literature. Choosing the most appropriate conversational strategy is an important consideration as this will determine the depth, breadth, and substance of the analysis. Eppich and Cheng (2015) divide conversational techniques into three main categories: (1) learner self-assessment strategies; (2) facilitated discussion strategies; and (3) directive feedback. We will review each in turn.

Learner Self-assessment

Using self-assessment strategies, facilitators can support learners to self-assess their own performance in the simulation activity. There are several strategies from which to choose. The most well-known, and most commonly, used is the Plus/Delta method. In this, the facilitator asks open-ended questions such as: "What went well?" or "What was easy?" (Plus) and "What could be changed?" or "What was challenging?" (Delta) (Fanning & Gaba, 2007). This strategy is relatively easy and straightforward for novice facilitators and can be useful in revealing the issues that are important to learners which can be probed using more directive methods later in the debrief.

Facilitated Discussions

Facilitator-guided discussion are the most commonly used method of post-event debriefing (Sawyer et al., 2016). One or more facilitators guide the conversation through the phases of the debrief and ensure that important learning points are covered. Learning points may be determined in advance and stated in the learning objectives, or they may be emergent – i.e. they are derived though actions and behaviours of the learners in the simulated event. Facilitated discussion promotes more in-depth analysis of events than would normally be achieved in a learner self-assessment approach. The facilitator can position themselves as a co-learner in the debrief, supporting learners to discover the frames and mental models that drove their actions. Alternatively, the facilitator can position themselves as a subject matter expert helping the learner to recognise flawed or faulty mental models and applying their knowledge and expertise to present alternative perspectives to the learners. Important learning will occur when facilitator and learners work together to develop alternative frames and actions for the future. One of the best known facilitated discussion techniques is Advocacy-Inquiry (Rudolph et al., 2006). This will be discussed in detail below in strategy 5.

Directive Feedback

It may be appropriate for facilitators to provide direct feedback to learners on their performance. Unlike the discussion-based approach described above, direct feedback tends to be a one-way communication of information to learners, and as such the facilitator's role is more like teaching than facilitating. Feedback can be seen as an efficient, clear and direct way to address a knowledge or performance gap that was identified in the simulation. The approach and methods of providing feedback vary widely and there is no best type of feedback for all learners or learning outcomes. Direct feedback has been shown to improve learning provided that learners are receptive and that the feedback is valid, objective, focused and clear (Shute, 2008).

Using a Blended Approach

Eppich and Cheng (2015) suggest that the blending of strategies to address given learning objectives may be appropriate. Consider a learning objective such as 'The team takes a structured approach to patient management'. In the analysis phase of the debrief the facilitator might first use self-assessment strategies, in order to discover what the learners found challenging about this activity. This may then be followed by a facilitated discussion to explore the frames that drove actions and, finally, directive feedback may be used to fill the learning need that has been identified. Eppich and Cheng (2015) present a framework called PEARLS (Promoting Excellence and Reflective Learning in Simulation) to guide the application for each of the three main strategies and to support facilitators in switching between strategies. The PEARLS approach also uses scripts to support the facilitator throughout the various stages of the debrief. Scripted debriefing will be discussed in more detail below in strategy 7.

STRATEGY 4: SELECT THE APPROPRIATE TIME POINT FOR THE DEBRIEF

Debriefing can occur either during the simulation event (within-event debriefing) or after the event (post-event debriefing). Within-event debriefing often involves strategies like "stop-action" debriefing where the facilitator stops the action and initiates a short conversation about actions taken (or not taken) and then starts the action again (Sawyer et al. 2016) This can be described as the *'pause and rewind and try again approach'*. This method is often used in association with rapid cycle deliberate practice (see Chapter 2). In post-event debriefing, the conversational structures and strategies described above are used to organise the debrief and achieve the learning objective through reflection and the analysis of events. This method is more commonly used in team simulations and simulation scenarios targeting non-technical skills such as teamwork, communication, or leadership.

STRATEGY 5: UTILISE SKILLED FACILITATORS

Debriefing by competent facilitators is considered important to maximise the learning arising from simulated events. There are several techniques that facilitators can employ to maximise engagement and learning from the debrief.

Ask Open-Ended Questions

Open questioning is a key skill of an effective facilitator (Sawyer et al., 2013; Kolbe et al., 2013). Asking open-ended questions helps facilitate discussion and foster reflection on the part of the learners. Examples of open-ended questions include: 'Can you tell me what happened during your telephone conversation with the consultant?' or 'Tell me about task allocation during the simulation.' Closed questions, which can be answered with 'Yes' or 'No', should be avoided as they do not generate discussion.

Use Silence

A period of silence can occur after a facilitator asks an open-ended question. Learners may need this time to process the question, reflect on their performance, and formulate a thoughtful response to the question. Therefore, facilitators must learn to allow this silence and avoid jumping in with their own thoughts, suggestions, and ideas (Ross, 2021). Silence will be more acceptable to learners if they are informed that some short periods of silence are to be expected during the debrief and that this time is for them to reflect and prepare their response.

Use Debriefing with Good Judgement

Another skill of experienced facilitators is the skill of disclosing judgements about learners' performance without being either too critical or too cryptic. Take the example of the debriefing question 'Were you well prepared for your conversation with the consultant?' Aside from the fact that it is a closed question, it also clearly has a judgement within it and the learner is left to guess what the judgement is. Rudolph et al., (2006) caution against this kind of questioning. Instead, they promote an approach to debriefing called 'debriefing with good judgement', which is presented as a way to debrief that brings forth the expert opinion of the facilitator, while, at the same time, it values the perspective of the learner. A particular conversational technique called Advocacy-Inquiry supports 'good judgement' questioning. Using Advocacy-Inquiry, the facilitator makes an observation and a judgement on a learner's action (Advocacy) and then inquires about the learner's frame of mind or reasons behind the action (Inquiry). An example of an Advocacy-Inquiry exchange may be something like this: "I noticed that you were leading the event but then you went to the phone to call for senior help" (observation); "I worried that taking on both tasks might compromise your ability to lead the event" (judgement); (observation + judgement = advocacy); "What was going through your mind when you decided to go to the phone" (Inquiry).

The basic stance of the facilitator during Advocacy-Inquiry is one of genuine curiosity. Actions, even those that are considered to be mistakes, are recognised to be the result of 'intentionally rational actions' (Rudolph et al., 2006). In other words, they made sense to the learner at the time given the how the learner was framing the situation:

> The debriefing with good judgement approach is designed to increase the chances that the trainee will be able to hear and process what the instructor is saying without being defensive or trying to guess what the instructor's critical judgement is.
>
> *(Rudolph et al., 2006)*

STRATEGY 6: CONSIDER IF VIDEO-ASSISTED DEBRIEFING (VAD) IS APPROPRIATE

Many larger simulation facilities, especially those that are purpose-built, have the potential to video-record the simulation event and use clips from the recording in the debrief in order to highlight particular aspects of performance. This is known as video-assisted debriefing (VAD) and it can be used to highlight areas of excellent or suboptimal performance. VAD is sometimes considered to be the 'gold standard' of debriefing. However, research evidence does not support the supposition. In fact, the use of VAD may not offer a significant advantage over verbal debriefing (Abeer & Miller,

2018; Wilbanks et al., 2020; Cheng et al., 2014). Similarly, evidence around learner and facilitator attitudes to VAD is also equivocal with some studies reporting positive attitudes to it and others negative attitudes (Zhang et al., 2019).

Krogh et al. (2015) conducted a study to explore expert facilitators' views on the use of VAD. The experts considered VAD to be an adjunct to debriefing rather than fundamental to it. They emphasised the need to balance the benefits and challenges of using VAD. The challenges were that technology may be a distraction to the facilitator and/or the learner, may disrupt the debriefing continuum, and may fail and derail the debrief. The identified benefits of VAD were that it aids learner recollection and learner reflection, triggers discussion, reduces the need to 'tell', and provides an objective perspective. To make VAD effective, specific educational techniques are thought to be required, including: informing learners of the educational purpose of viewing a clip; allowing time for learners to observe and reflect on their performance; allow learners time to self-evaluate their performance; providing examples of good practice; and using the clip as an instigator for discussion (Krogh et al., 2015).

Strategy 7: Consider Using Standardised or Scripted Debriefing

There is no doubt that debriefing can be daunting for novice facilitators. Part of the discomfort is derived from the fact that some of the learning points are emergent – arising from what actually transpired in the simulation. Thus, the facilitators must be able to think on their feet and juggle the predefined learning objective and the emergent agenda. While the learner may feel that they are in 'the spotlight' during the simulation, the facilitator may feel it is they who are in the spotlight during the debrief – especially if there are other faculty in the debrief. To support facilitators, particularly novice facilitators, Eppich and Cheng (2015) developed a structured framework known as PEARLS to provide a script for conducting a debriefing. There is some evidence to support the use of scripted debriefing over non-scripted debriefing with novice facilitators (Cheng et al., 2013). PEARLS directs facilitators to the most appropriate conversational strategy and includes scripts to guide the debrief. PEARLS supports the facilitator to:

- set the stage for the debriefing by providing a script for initiating the debriefing session to orientate the learner and tell them what is expected of them in the debrief;
- structure the debrief into four distinct phases: reactions, description, analysis, and summary; and
- select the most appropriate conversational strategy to use in the analysis phase and switch between strategies. Three screening questions help the facilitators to determine the ideal strategy to utilise for each learning objective or emergent learning point.
  1. Is there a clear performance gap?
  2. How much time is available?
  3. Does the performance represent cognitive, technical or behavioural domains?

(Eppich & Cheng, 2015)

DEBRIEFING AS FORMATIVE ASSESSMENT

As mentioned earlier, the debrief should be based on learning objectives that are specific, observable, achievable, appropriate, and easy to assess (see Chapter 3). These objectives are the standards of performance that learners are expected to achieve in their performance of the simulation. In the analysis phase of the debrief, learners' actual performance is compared against standards that were set out in the learning objectives. This process of comparing actual performance against a standard for the purpose of learning is a type of formative assessment. Formative assessment is discussed in more detail in the next chapter. However, it is also important to consider this form of assessment within the context of a debriefing. Rudolph et al. (2008) present a four-step model of debriefing as formative assessment:

1. note salient performance gaps related to predetermined objectives;
2. provide feedback describing the gap;

3. investigate the basis for the gap by exploring the frames and emotions contributing to the current performance level; and

4. help close the performance gap through discussion or targeted instruction about principles and skills relevant to performance.

DIFFICULT DEBRIEFING SITUATIONS

Debriefing can become strained for a number of reasons. Learners can derail the debrief by being reticent, overpowering, disengaged, defensive, emotional, or having poor insight. The debriefing situation can contribute to the problem, especially if the design and execution of the simulated event upset or troubled the learners in some way. An uncomfortable atmosphere in the debrief can be an indication that there is a mismatch between learner and facilitator perceptions and, if left unchecked, it can undermine the goals of the session and lead to a psychologically unsafe learning environment. Proactive strategies will be most effective in mitigating the risk of a difficult debrief. The prebrief is critical to set the expectations of the learners, establish an environment of mutual respect, establish a fiction contract, and set out the ground rules of the event (see Chapter 6 for more discussion). The approach that will be used in the debrief should also be described in the prebrief. In the debrief itself, creating an atmosphere that supports engagement and learning can be achieved by setting up the room in a way that is conducive to a conversation, reiterating the basic assumption and setting a tone that is respectful.

In terms of reactive strategies, Grant et al. (2018) identify seven approaches that can help to bring difficult debriefing conversations back on track. These strategies are summarised in Table 7.3

TABLE 7.3
Strategies to Manage Difficult Debriefing Situations

Strategy	Purpose	Example Wording
Normalisation	Signifies that the facilitator understands the learner's feelings and acknowledges that they are normal or common in these situations.	*"Other groups with similar experience level responded in the same way."* *"It is normal to feel overwhelmed in this situation."*
Validation	Signifies that the learners perspective is important.	*"I hear what you are saying, the composition of the team in the simulation was not the same as it is in normal practice."* *"I understand what you are saying; the manikin does not provide the same cues a patient would."*
Generalisation	Applying the experience to the real clinical context.	*"Has anyone experienced this in their practice?"* *"How might this manifest in clinical practice."*
Paraphrasing	Repeating what someone has said in your own words. It signals understanding or may help to clarify a point that a learner is making.	*"What I am hearing you say is that you believe that the manikin did not respond in the way that a 'normal' patient would given the actions that were taken and you found this frustrating…"*
Broadening	Widening the discussion to involve other learners. Brings in different perspectives and viewpoints. Can move the focus away from one learner.	*"I wonder what others think of this…?"* *"Has anyone else had a similar experience that they would like to share?"*
Previewing	The educator makes a statement to indicate the next topic for discussion.	*"I'd like to talk about task management for the next few minutes."* *"If it is OK with you I would like to change direction a bit and talk about the choice of medications."*
Naming the dynamic	Explicitly naming the emotion or energy in the room. Also known as 'stating the elephant in the room'.	*"I can see that this was really frustrating for you."* *"I can see that you are disappointed that you did not notice the clinical sign."*

Source: Adapted from Grant et al., 2018.

FACULTY TRAINING AND DEVELOPMENT

Given the importance of debriefing to learning in simulation, it is no surprise that facilitator training and development is an important consideration for simulation programmes. There is a relative paucity of guidance on the best methods to develop facilitator debriefing skills and facilitators tend to obtain debriefing training from various sources, including external courses, fellowships, through advanced degrees, workshops at conferences, and locally delivered courses such as 'train the trainer' courses. Formal faculty development is an option, and excellent training programmes exist internationally. However, formal training can be costly and, consequently, it is common for facilitators to have no formal training in debriefing (Cheng et al., 2016). Methods of faculty development that utilise the principles of peer coaching can be employed as an alternative to formal training, and it can be easier to integrate them into the daily activities (Cheng et al., 2017). "Encouraging faculty to provide colleagues with constructive feedback forms the foundation for a culture of transparency, teamwork, and patient safety that ultimately results in the delivery of higher-quality healthcare" (Cheng et al., 2017: 320). One commonly used strategy that utilises the principles of peer coaching is 'debriefing the debrief'.

'DEBRIEFING THE DEBRIEF'

The term 'debriefing the debrief' is used to describe the process of reviewing a debrief in order to assess its effectiveness and identify areas for improvement. Recognising the value of this improvement mindset, the team of simulation educators at the National Health Service (NHS) Lothian in Scotland initiated a 'debriefing the debrief' programme called 'The Meta-Debrief Club' or MDC. It was recognised that although debriefers may have many opportunities to practice, practice alone will not necessarily improve performance unless it is combined with focused reflection to drive improvement. To this end, the MDC took part in a regular evaluation of their practice, with constructive feedback from peers (O'Shea et al., 2020). It is interesting to note that the same principles and practices that the educators use to enhance *student* learning was also applied to the debriefers in order to improve *their own* performance. The strategy employed for MDC sessions involved showing video footage of a debrief session followed by a discussion which utilises much the same strategies as was used in the debrief itself, i.e. lead facilitator explores the facilitator's frames or mental models, learning points are identified and take-home messages or changes the facilitator will incorporate into their practice are determined. As with all debriefing, careful consideration is given to maintaining participants' psychological safety during the process. Debriefing the debrief can be facilitated when a structured approach is taken with the appraisal of the debrief. Two appraisal tools are widely cited in the research literature. These are described below.

THE OBSERVATIONAL STRUCTURED ASSESSMENT OF DEBRIEFING TOOL (OSAD)

The OSAD is an observation tool that provides a structured framework for evaluating the key elements of a debriefing session *and* the facilitators' performance in that session (Runnacles et al., 2014; Imperial College London, 2012). The OSAD tool was originally developed for paediatric simulation debriefing but has application to any area of healthcare simulation debriefing. For example, this tool was used to guide the feedback in the MDC described above (O'Shea et al., 2020).

The OSAD tool identifies eight core components of effective debriefing that were identified via literature review and expert opinion: (1) facilitators' approach; (2) learning environment; (3) engagement of learners; (4) reaction; (5) reflection; (6) analysis; (7) diagnosis; and (8) application to future practice. Table 7.4 provides an overview of the OSAD rating scale. The OSAD provides a standardised method for evaluating the effectiveness of debriefing sessions.

TABLE 7.4
The OSAD Rating Scale

Element	Level 1	Level 2	Level 3	Level 4	Level 5
Facilitators' approach	Confrontational/ judgemental approach.				Establishes rapport, creates a non-threatening environment, establishes psychological safety.
Learning environment	Unclear expectations and inadequate environment.				Explains purpose, objectives and expectations.
Engagement of learners	Didactic style, no learner engagement.				Encourages participation, invites contribution, uses open-ended questions.
Reaction	No acknowledgement of learner emotions.				Fully explores learners' reactions and manages emotions appropriately.
Descriptive reflection	No opportunity for self-reflection.				Encourages self-reflection.
Analysis	Reasons and consequences not explored.				Helps learners explore reasons and consequences and relates learning to previous experience.
Diagnosis	Does not identify performance gaps or provide positive reinforcement.				Identifies positive behaviours in addition to performance gaps.
Application to future practice	No opportunity to identify strategies for improvement.				Reinforces key learning points and highlights application to future practice.

Sources: Adapted from Imperial College London, 2012.

DEBRIEFING ASSESSMENT FOR SIMULATION IN HEALTHCARE (DASH)

Another tool that is used to assess the effectiveness of debriefing sessions following a SBE is the DASH tool (Brett-Fleegler et al., 2012). Similar to the OSAD, DASH utilises a behaviourally anchored rating scale to assess what instructors do or fail to do. Unlike the OSAD, the DASH tool can be used to assess the prebrief and the debrief. The DASH has six elements which are rated on a 7-point behaviourally anchored rating scale, ranging from 1 (extremely ineffective/detrimental) to 7 (extremely effective/outstanding). Table 7.5 provides an overview of the DASH rating scale.

Both the DASH and the OSAD provide a common language for desirable debrief process and practices. For this reason, these tools can be used to assess the debriefing strategy used (either generally or, more specifically, within a specific SBE event) and also the skills of the facilitator. This information can be used to provide structured feedback to faculty in the context of a peer-coaching process.

TABLE 7.5

The DASH Elements and Dimensions

Dash Element	Element Dimensions
Establishes an engaging learning environment	• Clarifies objectives, roles, and expectations. • Establishes a 'fiction contract' with participants. • Attends to logistic details. • Conveys a commitment to respecting learners.
Maintains an engaging learning environment	• Clarifies debriefing objectives, roles, and expectations. • Helps participants engage with the simulation context. • Conveys respect for learners and concern for their psychological safety.
Structures the debriefing in an organised way	• Encourages learners to express their reactions. • Orients learners to what happened in the simulation. • Guides analysis of the learners' performance. • Collaborates with participants to summarise learning.
Provokes engaging discussions	• Uses concrete examples as the basis for inquiry and discussion. • Reveals own reasoning and judgements. • Facilitates discussion through verbal and non-verbal techniques. • Uses video, replay, and review devices (if available). • Recognises and manages the upset learner.
Identifies and explores performance gaps	• Provides feedback on performance. • Explores the source of the performance gap.
Helps learners achieve or sustain good future performance	• Helps close the performance gap through discussion and teaching. • Demonstrates firm grasp of the subject. • Meets the important objectives of the session.

Source: Adapted from Brett-Fleegler et al., 2012.

CONCLUSION

Debriefing should be the cornerstone of SBE (Husebø et al., 2015). It is the process through which learners reflect upon the experience that has occurred in a simulated event. Although there are many approaches to debriefing, there are also broad commonalities across these different methods. Whatever debriefing approach is used, it is recommended that a simulation facility should have a debriefing "house style". Such standardisation in debriefing practices will ensure that the facilitators develop expertise in using this style, meaning that facilitators can easily swap between different SBE activities at the facility, and ensures that faculty and learners are habituated to how debriefing is carried out at the facility. However, whatever specific approach is chosen for debriefing in a facility, the facilitator must have the flexibility to allow the debriefing to be aligned to the learning needs, the learning context, the objectives of the session, the experience of the learners, and the skills of the facilitator.

FURTHER READING

Barry Issenberg, S., McGaghie, W. C., Petrusa, E. R., Lee Gordon, D., Scalese, R. J. (2005). Features and uses of high-fidelity medical simulations that lead to effective learning, a BEME systematic review. *Medical Teacher, 27*(1), 10–28.

Brett-Fleegler, M., Rudolph, J., Eppich, W., Monuteaux, M., Fleegler, E., Cheng, A., Simon, R. (2012). Debriefing assessment for simulation in healthcare, development and psychometric properties. *Simulation in Healthcare, 7*(5), 288–294.

Eppich, W., Cheng, A. (2015). Promoting Excellence and Reflective Learning in Simulation (PEARLS), development and rationale for a blended approach to health care simulation debriefing. *Simulation in Healthcare, 10*(2), 106–115.

Motola, I., Devine, L. A., Chung, H. S., Sullivan, J. E., Issenberg, S. B. (2013). Simulation in healthcare education, a best evidence practical guide. AMEE Guide No. 82. *Medical Teacher*, *35*(10),142–159.

Purva, M., Nicklin, J. (2018). ASPiH standards for simulation-based education, process of consultation, design and implementation. *BMJ Simulation & Technology Enhanced Learning*, *4*(3), 117.

Raemer, D., Anderson, M., Cheng, A., Fanning, R., Nadkarni, V., Savoldelli, G. (2011). Research regarding debriefing as part of the learning process. *Simulation in Healthcare*, *6*(7), S52–S57.

Rudolph, J. W., Simon, R., Dufresne, R. L., Raemer, D. B. (2006). There's no such thing as "nonjudgmental" debriefing, a theory and method for debriefing with good judgment. *Simulation in Healthcare*, *1*(1), 49–55.

Rudolph, J. W., Simon, R., Raemer, D. B., Eppich, W. J. (2008). Debriefing as formative assessment, closing performance gaps in medical education. *Academic Emergency Medicine*, *15*(11), 1010–1016.

ONLINE RESOURCES

- ASPiH Standards for Simulation-Based Education (SBE): aspih.org.uk/standards-framework-for-sbe/.
- ASPiH Standards Framework: aspih.org.uk/wp-content/uploads/2017/07/standards-framework.pdf.
- Information on the OSAD tool: www.imperial.ac.uk/patient-safety-translational-research-centre/education/training-materials-for-use-in-research-and-clinical-practice/the-observational-structured/.
- Information on the DASH tool: https://harvardmedsim.org/debriefing-assessment-for-simulation-in-healthcare-dash/
- Society for Simulation in Healthcare: www.ssih.org/About-SSH/About-Simulation.

REFERENCES

Abeer, A. A., Miller, E. T. (2018). Effectiveness of video-assisted debriefing in health education, an integrative review. *Journal of Nursing Education*, *57*(1), 14–20.

Brett-Fleegler, M., Rudolph, J., Eppich, W., Monuteaux, M., Fleegler, E., Cheng, A., Simon, R. (2012). Debriefing assessment for simulation in healthcare, development and psychometric properties. *Simulation in Healthcare*, *7*(5), 288–294.

Cheng, A., Eppich, W., Grant, V., Sherbino, J., Zendejas, B., Cook, D. A. (2014). Debriefing for technology-enhanced simulation, a systematic review and meta-analysis. *Medical Education*, *48*(7), 657–666.

Cheng, A., Hunt, E. A., Donoghue, A., Nelson-McMillan, K., Nishisaki, A., LeFlore, J., Eppich, W., Moyer, M., Brett-Fleegler, M., Kleinman, M., Anderson, J. (2013). Examining pediatric resuscitation education using simulation and scripted debriefing, a multicenter randomized trial. *JAMA Pediatrics*, *167*(6), 528–536.

Cheng, A., Grant, V., Robinson, T., Catena, H., Lachapelle, K., Kim, J., Eppich, W. (2016). The Promoting Excellence and Reflective Learning in Simulation (PEARLS) approach to health care debriefing, a faculty development guide. *Clinical Simulation in Nursing*, *12*(10), 419–428.

Cheng, A., Grant, V., Huffman, J., Burgess, G., Szyld, D., Robinson, T., Eppich, W. (2017). Coaching the facilitator, peer coaching to improve debriefing quality in simulation programs. *Simulation in Healthcare*, *12*(5), 319–325.

Eppich, W., Cheng, A. (2015). Promoting Excellence and Reflective Learning in Simulation (PEARLS), development and rationale for a blended approach to health care simulation debriefing. *Simulation in Healthcare*, *10*(2), 106–115.

Fanning, R. M., Gaba, D. M. (2007). The role of debriefing in simulation-based learning. *Simulation in Healthcare*, *2*(2), 115–125.

Grant, V. J., Robinson, T., Catena, H., Eppich, W., Cheng, A. (2018). Difficult debriefing situations, a toolbox for simulation educators. *Medical Teacher*, *40*(7), 703–712.

Husebø, S. E., O'Regan, S., Nestel, D. (2015). Reflective practice and its role in simulation. *Clinical Simulation in Nursing*, *11*(8), 368–375.

Imperial College, London. (2012). *The London Handbook for Debriefing: Enhancing Debriefing in Clinical and Simulated Settings*. London: Imperial College.

INACSL Standards Committee. (2016). INACSL standards of best practice, simulation debriefing. *Clinical Simulation in Nursing*, *12*, S21–S25.

Jaye, P., Thomas, L., Reedy, G. (2015). 'The Diamond', a structure for simulation debrief. *Clinical Teacher*, *12*(3), 171–175.

Kolb, D. A. (1984). *Experiential Learning: Experience as the Source of Learning and Development*. Englewook Cliffs, NJ: Prentice-Hall.

Kolbe, M., Weiss, M., Grote, G., Knauth, A., Dambach, M., Spahn, D. R., Grande, B. (2013). TeamGAINS, a tool for structured debriefings for simulation-based team trainings. *BMJ Quality & Safety*, *22*(7), 541–553.

Krogh, K., Bearman, M., Nestel, D. (2015). Expert practice of video-assisted debriefing, an Australian qualitative study. *Clinical Simulation in Nursing*, *11*(3), 180–187.

Lioce, L., et al. (Eds.). (2020). *Healthcare Simulation Dictionary - Second Edition*. Rockville, MD: Agency for Healthcare Research and Quality.

Motola, I., Devine, L. A., Chung, H. S., Sullivan, J. E., Issenberg, S. B. (2013). Simulation in healthcare education: a best evidence practical guide. AMEE Guide No. 82. *Medical Teacher*, *35*(10),142–159.

O'Shea, C. I., Schnieke-Kind, C., Pugh, D., Picton, E. (2020). The Meta-Debrief Club: an effective method for debriefing your debrief. *BMJ Simulation & Technology Enhanced Learning*, *6*(2), 118–120.

Phrampus, P. E., O'Donnell, J. M. (2013). Debriefing using a structured and supported approach. In: Levine, A. I., DeMaria, S., Schwartz, A. D., Sim, A. J. (Eds.) *The Comprehensive Textbook of Healthcare Simulation* (pp. 73–84). New York: Springer.

Ross, S. (2021). Twelve tips for effective simulation debriefing, a research-based approach. *Medical Teacher*, *43*(6), 642–645.

Rudolph, J. W., Simon, R., Raemer, D. B., Eppich, W. J. (2008). Debriefing as formative assessment, closing performance gaps in medical education. *Academic Emergency Medicine*, *15*(11), 1010–1016.

Rudolph, J. W., Simon, R., Dufresne, R. L., Raemer, D. B. (2006). There's no such thing as "nonjudgmental" debriefing, a theory and method for debriefing with good judgment. *Simulation in Healthcare*, *1*(1), 49–55.

Runnacles, J., Thomas, L., Sevdalis, N., Kneebone, R., Arora, S., Cooper, M. (2014). Development of a tool to improve performance debriefing and learning: the paediatric Objective Structured Assessment of Debriefing (OSAD) tool. *Postgraduate Medical Journal*, *90*(1069), 613–621.

Sawyer, T., Eppich, W., Brett-Fleegler, M., Grant, V., Cheng, A. (2016). More than one way to debrief: a critical review of healthcare simulation debriefing methods. *Simulation in Healthcare*, *11*(3), 209–217.

Schön, D. A. (2017). *The Reflective Practitioner: How Professionals Think in Action*. Milton Park, UK: Routledge.

Shute, V. J. (2008). Focus on formative feedback. *Review of Educational Research*, *78*(1), 153–189.

Wilbanks, B. A., McMullan, S., Watts, P. I., White, T., Moss, J. (2020). Comparison of video-facilitated reflective practice and faculty-led debriefings. *Clinical Simulation in Nursing*, *42*, 1–7.

Zhang, H., Mörelius, E., Goh, S. H. L., Wang, W. (2019). Effectiveness of video-assisted debriefing in simulation-based health professions education, a systematic review of quantitative evidence. *Nurse Educator*, *44*(3), E1–E6.

8 Assessment

KEY POINTS

- Given the strong relationship between assessment and learning it is important that careful consideration is given to what is assessed in a simulation-based education (SBE), as well as how this should be carried out.
- Assessment can be either formative or summative. Formative assessment is a low-stakes process with a focus on improvement. It tends to occur throughout the learning period. Summative assessment, by contrast, generally occurs at the end of a period of learning. The focus of summative assessment is on accessing whether a standard of performance is achieved in order to allow the learner to advance to the next level of training or education.
- The goal of assessment should be to determine the strengths and weaknesses of the learners – achieving this will require the integration of formative and summative assessment.
- There are four criteria to consider when determining the usefulness of a particular method of assessment: reliability; validity; feasibility; and educational impact.
- Assessment should be supported by an appropriate assessment framework – this can be an assessment checklist, a global rating system, or both.
- We, as simulationists, must become more comfortable with assessment of our own teaching.

INTRODUCTION

A common adage in medical education is Miller's (1990) assertion that *'assessment drives learning'*. This phrase is often taken to mean that learners will focus on what will be assessed. However, it can also mean that assessment can be considered a part of the learning process. Miller (1990) suggests that assessment drives learning in four ways: (1) in the content of the learning; (2) the timing of the learning; (3) the format of the learning; and (4) the feedback provided. Seen in this way, assessment can have a powerful influence on what is taught, how it is taught, when it is taught, and the nature of the feedback. Learning outcomes have a clear role to play in this dynamic. In fact, Biggs (2003) introduces the idea of constructive alignment to conceptualise the relationship between learning outcomes, content (learning activity), and assessment. Constructive alignment simply means that the learning activity and assessment are aligned to the predefined learning outcomes. The role of feedback is also recognised as critical in the assessment–learning relationship. Brown and Pickford (2006) describe feedback as the "oil which lubricates the engine of learning". Given a strong relationship between assessment and learning it is important that careful consideration is given to what is assessed and how the assessment is undertaken.

DOI: 10.1201/9781003296942-8

CHAPTER OVERVIEW

This chapter will:

- outline formative and summative assessment;
- discuss the criteria to be considered when determining the usefulness of a particular method of assessment;
- describe two different types of assessment frameworks suitable for assessing procedural and nontechnical skills; and
- identify approaches to assessing simulation educators.

ASSESSMENT

Assessment is concerned with evaluating whether a learner has achieved a predetermined standard of performance. There are many ways to assess performance and there is increasing recognition that simulation offers the opportunity for the authentic and realistic assessment of practical skills. The outputs of the assessment will depend on the goal of the assessment; if the goal is for learning and improvement, the outcome of the assessment will be feedback and possible remediation. If the goal is for evaluation, the output will be a grade or rating that will be used to determine whether the learner has achieved the level of performance that is required. Epstein (2007) identifies three main goals of assessment in medical education: (1) to optimise the capabilities of learners by providing motivation and direction for future learning; (2) to protect patients by identifying incompetent healthcare practitioners; and (3) to provide a basis for choosing applicants for advanced training.

FORMATIVE AND SUMMATIVE ASSESSMENT

Assessment can be either formative or summative. Formative assessment is usually a low-stakes process with a focus on giving feedback to the learner on how they are progressing. As such, the purpose of formative assessment is to encourage self-reflection by the learner, and to identify areas of strength and weakness in performance. In contrast, summative assessment is usually high-stakes. Summative assessment generally occurs at the end of a period of learning in which the achievement of a predetermined standard of performance is required in order to advance to the next level of training or education. For this reason, for summative assessment, it is particularly important that there are clear learning objectives which set out the expected standards in a measurable way (see Chapter 3).

The methods of assessment suitable for formative and summative assessment may not be the same. As the goal of formative assessment is to promote learner self-reflection and improvement, formative assessment can be likened to a debriefing. Indeed, in the previous chapter we discussed debriefing as a form of formative assessment where a learner's performance is assessed against a standard of performance (as outlined in the learning objectives) and this comparison, and also the discussion that surrounds it, is an important part of the learning from the activity. In contrast, as the focus of summative assessment is on readiness for advancement, there is a need to ensure that the summative assessment is of sufficient validity and reliability for high-stakes evaluation. While the focus of summative assessment is usually on evaluation, the process can also be designed to generate feedback for the learner which can be useful in driving learning (Schuwirth & Van der Vleuten, 2004).

Traditionally, in healthcare education, there has been a focus on summative assessment. However, this is beginning to change. The goal of assessment should be to determine the strengths and weaknesses of the learners to optimise their individual learning pathways (Schuwirth & Van der Vleuten, 2004). Achieving this goal will require the integration of formative and summative assessment. Also, although the focus of assessment is usually on the performance of the learner, it can also be used as an assessment of the teaching. If the assessment identifies that learners are not achieving the desired standard of performance, there may be a need to review the teaching as well as the standard of performance.

OBJECTIVE STRUCTURED CLINICAL EXAMINATION (OSCE)

One common form of summative assessments using healthcare simulation are Objective Structured Clinical Examinations (OSCEs). OSCEs were first described by Harden et al. (1975). An OSCE evaluates a learner's ability to perform a particular clinical task (e.g. to complete a physical exam).

An OSCE usually consists of a circuit of short stations (each of which is 8 to 10 minutes in length). At each station, the learner is assessed on their performance of a particular clinical task by an examiner who observes their performance. An OCSE station may require the performance of a clinical procedural task using a simulator or task trainer, or it may involve an interaction with a simulated participant (SP), or both. The learners complete a number of stations in an OSCE circuit. An OSCE is objective because all of the learners are assessed performing the same stations with the same scoring rubric. It is also structured because there are specific objectives that a learner is expected to achieve at each station, with careful scripting to ensure that the task, including any interactions with SPs, are standardised for each learner. Thirdly, it is a clinical exam because the focus is on assessing the application of clinical skills and knowledge. OSCEs can be used for formative or summative assessment. They also allow an assessment to be made of a learner's technical and nontechnical skills (e.g. communication), or both.

DETERMINING THE USEFULNESS OF ASSESSMENT

Van der Vleuten and Schuwirth (2005) identify four criteria for determining the usefulness of a particular method of assessment: (1) reliability; (2) validity, (3) feasibility; and (4) educational impact. Whole books could be written on each one of these topics. Our aim in this chapter is to introduce these criteria and explain why they are important considerations when using simulation for assessment. These criteria will be discussed within the context of an OSCE – as this is a common form of simulation-based assessment.

RELIABILITY

Reliability is concerned with the reproducibility of the assessment. Although still relevant, reliability is of less concern for formative assessment, but is very important for high-stakes summative assessment. A very reliable assessment will mean that all learners at the same level of ability will receive the same score for their performance on the assessment. This is obviously especially important in a high-stakes assessment. It is beyond the scope of this chapter, but there are a range of metrics than can be used to evaluate the reliability of OSCEs (e.g. *Cronbach's α* or *G coefficient*). These metrics can be used post-hoc to identify if there are issues with the reliability of a particular station or examiner. This information can then be used to adjust the scores of the learners in high-stakes OSCEs to improve the reliability of the assessment. Pell et al. (2010) provide and excellent review of a range of metrics for assessing the reliability of OSCEs. If these metrics are to be used to adjust scores in a high-stakes assessment, then it is important that there is input from a statistician. However, rather than attempting to 'fix' issues with reliability after an OSCE has been completed, it is preferable to take measures to ensure that that an OSCE is reliable before it is run. Khan et al. (2013b) identify four approaches to increasing the reliability of an OSCE:

- *Use multiple OSCE stations and blueprint against the curriculum.* Typically, a final-year medical school OSCE consists of between 10 and 20 individual stations (Gormley, 2011). A larger number of OSCE stations generates greater reliability than a smaller number of stations. This makes sense in that many stations evens out the effect of an unusually good (or poor) performance by a learner or the effect of a harsh or lenient examiner at one particular station. Clearly, OSCE stations should assess what has been covered in the curriculum and match what learners should be expected to achieve at their level of progression.

- *Use a standardised scoring rubric.* To support consistency in the assessment of learners, examiners require clear criteria for various levels of performance. This is discussed in more detail later in the chapter within the context of assessment frameworks.
- *Train examiners.* Research suggests that examiners that have not received training are less consistent and more lenient than trained examiners (Pell et al., 2008). Khan et al. (2013a) suggest that on completion of the training, the examiner should:
  - understand the scope and principles of the OSCE examination;
  - understand how to behave professionally during the examination;
  - understand and use the scoring rubric consistently;
  - know how to provide written feedback on performance in summative examinations (if required);
  - know how to provide verbal feedback at the end of a station in formative examinations;
  - ensure the confidentiality of the learners' assessment sheets; and
  - understand the procedures for inappropriate or dangerous behaviour by learners.
- *Train Simulated Participants (SPs).* It is important that if SPs are used in an OSCE station they are also trained to ensure that that there is consistency in their performance between the different learners. It may take considerable practice and feedback to ensure that an actor is delivering a consistent performance. It has been suggested that it may take 15 hours to adequately train a SP – depending on the role, level of experience and adaptability of the actor (Shumway & Harden, 2003). Moreover, increasingly SPs are being used to provide feedback to learners in formative and summative assessments – particularly with respect to the interpersonal skills of the learner. If this is the case, as with the examiners, the SPs will need to be provided with training on how to deliver feedback to the learners.

VALIDITY

Validity is concerned with whether the assessment measures what it intends to measure. It is important to draw a distinction between validity and reliability. An assessment may be reliable, with consistency across examiners, SPs, etc. However, the assessment could still be invalid. For example, an assessment of how to perform a procedure based upon an outdated protocol.

There are many different types of validity. However, *content validity* is particularly important for OSCEs. Content validity is concerned with the extent to which the OSCE assessment matches the learning outcomes and the learning activity within the course of instruction (Gormley, 2011). It relates to the constructive alignment between the educational outcomes, the learning activity, and the assessment. This determination can be made through a process known as blueprinting in which the content of an assessment is formally determined (Gormley, 2011; Khan et al., 2013a). Blueprinting ensures that the learning objectives and outcomes of an educational intervention are addressed in the assessment. There is also a need to consider whether a particular learning outcome is assessed in more than one way (e.g. assessing both verbal and written communication).

FEASIBILITY

The feasibility of an OSCE is an important consideration. Compromise may be required between what is ideal versus what is practical. By way of illustration, we recently ran an OSCE circuit for junior doctors to evaluate performance of nine basic clinical procedures. It took approximately three hours for each participant to rotate through all nine assessments and required an assessor (or examiner) for each procedure. To evaluate 10 junior doctors requires around 100 person hours (25 person-hours to set-up/tear down of the simulators, 37.5 person-hours for the junior doctors to participate in the assessment, and 37.5 hours for the assessors). This calculation does not include the time taken to design the OSCE stations and assessments, the administration in terms of room bookings and ensuring the participants and assessors show up at the correct time/place, nor collating and analysing the performance. Therefore, it is important to ensure that the best use possible is made of an OSCE assessment. OSCEs should be used to assess skills, or behaviours, that cannot be assessed in any other way. OSCE should not be used to assess knowledge which can assessed in less labour-intensive ways (Khan et al., 2013). Moreover, learners should receive feedback on their performance to capitalise on the opportunities for learning from the event.

EDUCATIONAL IMPACT

The impact of the OSCE should be beyond the passing or failing of an examination, and in an ideal world the assessment will drive life-long learning. If this goal is to be achieved, it is important that the assessment relates to the activities and the skills required in the actual clinical environment. This relatedness to the clinical environment is concerned with the realism, or fidelity, of the simulation (discussed in Chapter 1). Arguably, the most important dimension to address in an OSCE is the psychological fidelity or realism. That is, the extent to which the simulation mimics the psychological and cognitive factors that are present in the real clinical environment such that the learner suspends disbelief and interacts in the simulation as they would in the real clinical environment. If high psychological realism or fidelity can be achieved, then this will extend the educational impact of the assessment beyond the passing or failing of the exam.

ASSESSMENT FRAMEWORKS

As discussed above, an assessment framework, such as a standardised scoring rubric, supports an assessor to reliably assess the performance of a learner, and to provide structured feedback on the performance of the learner. Below we will discuss approaches to assessing procedural and nontechnical skills.

ASSESSING PROCEDURAL SKILLS

As discussed in Chapter 2, clear criteria for performing a procedure are fundamental to behaviour-based approaches to teaching such as deliberate practice and precision teaching. Direct observation of procedural skills (DOPS) is one common approach used to evaluate performance of a procedural skill. The learner (in either a simulated or a real clinical setting) is observed performing the skill and assessed using a checklist to record whether the steps in the procedure have been performed correctly (see Example 8.1).

Often, in addition to the checklist assessment, the assessor also provides a global rating of the learner's performance of the procedure or task. To illustrate, for Example 8.1, in addition to identifying whether the individual steps were correctly performed, the assessor could also provide a broad assessment of holistic aspects of the learner's performance (i.e., poor, marginal, acceptable, or good). For high-stakes testing, utilising both the checklist and the global rating is preferable as it allows for an assessment of the quality of a particular OSCE station. For example, if the checklist ratings are high, indicating that the candidate performed the steps correctly, but the global ratings are low, then this is an indication that there is a mismatch between what is on the checklist and what is required in a competent performance of the task. (for more discussion see Pell et al., 2010).

There are advantages and disadvantages in the use of both checklists and global rating scales for assessing performance. Checklists are generally easy to use and provide a clear outline of the steps.

EXAMPLE 8.1   CHECKLIST FOR THE ASSESSMENT OF VENEPUNCTURE SKILL

Checklist rating.

1. Label bottles and fill out laboratory request forms
2. Perform hand hygiene
3. Clean tray
4. Open equipment
5. Perform hand hygiene
6. Apply gloves
7. Apply tourniquet
8. Palpate a suitable vein
9. Cleanse skin
10. Relax tourniquet, and all alcohol to dry
11. Re-apply tourniquet
12. Unsheath needle

13. Insert needle, bevel up
14. Fill bottles in correct sequence (order of the draw)
15. Release tourniquet
16. Deploy needle safety, remove needle, & apply pressure
17. Place blood bottle in lab request bag
18. Apply strip plaster
19. Dispose of all waste
20. Remove gloves, dispose in clinical waste
21. Perform hand hygiene

(completed, partially completed, or not done)

Source: Reid-McDermott et al., 2022.

Therefore, even someone who is not particularly familiar with the procedure can evaluate the performance of the learner (Ilgen et al., 2015). A checklist also helps in providing feedback to a learner as to where they have not completed a step correctly. However, checklists must be developed for each specific procedure. It is also necessary to establish an agreed 'correct way' to complete a task, and complex tasks may require an exceptionally lengthy list of steps.

Global rating scales allow the assessor to provide feedback on issues that may not be captured in a checklist, and so better capture "nuanced elements of expertise" than checklists (Ilgen et al., 2015). Global ratings can be used across multiple procedures and negate the need for every step in the procedure to be delineated and assessed. However, the assessor must be very familiar with the procedure, and there is a reliance upon an expert assessment that may bring the defensibility of a high-stakes assessment into question (Ilgen et al., 2015). It has also been suggested that more training is required to use a global rating scale reliably as compared to a checklist (Ilgen et al., 2015). Neither checklists nor global ratings are 'better' assessments than the other. If used correctly, both demonstrate good reliability (Ilgen et al., 2015). The most important consideration is that no matter what method of evaluation is used, the assessment is consistent with how the procedure was taught to the learner.

A particular global rating, called the Objective Structured Assessment of Technical Skills (OSATS) system, developed for surgical procedures is shown in Example 8.2. It can be seen that the OSATS global rating system could be applied to any surgical procedure. There is validity evidence to support the use of the OSATS for formative feedback (Hatala et al., 2015), and high levels of inter-rater reliability have been reported when OSATS is used by experienced assessors (Chang et al., 2016).

Assessing Non-technical Skills

Non-technical skills (NTS) can be defined as the social (e.g. teamwork, leadership, communication), cognitive (e.g. situation awareness, decision-making,) and self- management (e.g. stress and fatigue management) skills necessary for safe and effective performance (Flin et al., 2008). In well-bounded simulation activity, such as an OSCE station involving an SP encounter, it is usually possible to

EXAMPLE 8.2   OBJECTIVE STRUCTURED ASSESSMENT OF TECHNICAL SKILLS (OSATS)

	1	2	3	4	5
Respect for tissue	Frequently used unnecessary force on tissue or caused damage by inappropriate use of instrument.		Careful handling of tissue, but occasionally caused inadvertent damage.		Consistently handled tissues appropriately with minimal damage.
Time and motion	Many unnecessary moves.		Efficient time/motion but some unnecessary moves.		Economy of movement with maximum efficiency.
Instrument handling	Repeatedly makes tentative or awkward moves with instruments.		Competent use of instruments, although occasional awkwardness.		Fluid moves with instruments and no awkwardness.
Knowledge of instruments	Frequently asked for the wrong instrument or used an inappropriate instrument.		Knew the name of most instruments and used appropriate instruments for the task.		Obvious familiarity with the required instruments and their names.
Use of assistants	Consistently placed assistants poorly or failed to use assistants.		Good use of assistants most of the time.		Strategic use of assistants to the best advantage at all times.
Flow of operation & forward planning	Frequently stopped operating or needed to discuss next move.		Demonstrated ability for forward planning with steady progression of operative procedure.		Obviously planned course of operation with effortless flow from one move to the next.
Knowledge of specific procedure	Deficient knowledge. Needed specific instruction at most operative steps.		Knew all important aspects of the procedure.		Demonstrated familiarity with all aspects of the procedure.

Source: Adapted from Martin et al., 1997.

develop a checklist to assess the required NTS – see Example 8.3. However, the assessment of NTS can be challenging for more complex scenarios such as an assessment of a trauma team. In a healthcare team the performance of any individual is dependent on other team members and so there tends to be more variability in how a scenario may progress. Thus, it may not be possible to use a checklist because there is not an ordered list of clearly defined behaviours or activities. Therefore, for these types of complex scenarios a more global approach to assessment is appropriate such as a behavioural marker system.

Behavioural markers. Behavioural markers are a structured observational system to supports the assessment of observable NTS that contribute to superior or substandard performance (Flin et al., 2008). A good behavioural marker describes a specific, observable behaviour, rather than an attitude or personality trait and has a clear definition. The behaviour should have a demonstrated causal relationship to performance outcome. It also does not have to be present in every scenario.

EXAMPLE 8.3   CHECKLIST FOR THE ASSESSMENT OF A PATIENT COMMUNICATION OSCE STATION

Checklist rating (completed, partially completed, not done)

Initiate the consultation
1. Introduces self and role and greets patient.
2. Outlines the purpose of the consultation and gives an overview of what will be discussed.
3. Assesses the patient's starting point.

Build the relationship
4. Listens attentively, minimising interruption and leaving space for replies.
5. Demonstrates appropriate non-verbal behaviour e.g. eye contact.
6. Uses empathy.

Aiding accurate recall and understanding
7. Structures the consultation in a logical sequence.
8. Chunks information and checks the individual's understanding.
9. Uses plain language, avoids jargon and confusing language.

Achieving a shared understanding: incorporating the other individual's perspective
10. Progresses from one section to another using signposting; includes rationale for next section.
11. Encourages individuals to contribute reactions, feelings and own ideas.
12. Picks up and responds to verbal and non-verbal cues, e.g. facial expression.

Shared decision-making, planning and closure
13. Explores management options with the patient.
14. Appropriately negotiates mutually acceptable action plan.
15. Summarises session consultation and care plan.

An example of a behavioural marker system designed for anaesthesiologists (ANTS) is shown in Example 8.4, and a system for scrub practitioners (SPLINTS) in Example 8.5. It can be seen that the behavioural marker system consists of behaviour categories, which are subdivided into more specific behavioural elements. An assessor rates the candidate on each category and element. For ANTS and SPLINTS, the possible ratings are:

- *Good* – performance was of a consistently high standard, enhancing patient safety; it could be used as a positive example for others.
- *Acceptable* – performance was of a satisfactory standard but could be improved.
- *Marginal* – performance indicated cause for concern, considerable improvement is needed.
- *Poor* – performance endangered or potentially endangered patient safety, serious remediation is required.
- *Not-observed* – skill was not observed in this situation (Mitchell et al., 2013).

Behavioural marker systems are context-specific, and are developed for the domain in which they are to be used (Flin et al., 2008). However, if you compare across behavioural marker systems in different domains of healthcare (e.g. anaesthesiology, surgery), and even those developed for use in other high-risk domains (e.g. civil aviation, Flin et al., 2018; military ships, O'Connor & Long, 2011), there are commonalities across the systems – particularly at the category level. This makes intuitive sense in that NTS such as communication or situation awareness are just as important for a surgeon as they are for the officer-of-the-deck responsible for manoeuvring a large warship in a congested harbour.

There is some evidence to support the reliability and validity of behavioural marker systems described in the research literature (Dietz et al., 2014). As with the assessment of clinical procedural

EXAMPLE 8.4   ANAESTHETIST NONTECHNICAL SKILLS (ANTS)

Category	Element
Task management	• Planning and preparing management • Prioritising • Providing and maintaining standards • Identifying and utilising resources
Teamworking	• Coordinating activities with team members • Exchanging information • Using authority and assertiveness • Assessing capabilities • Supporting others
Situation awareness	• Gathering information • Recognising and understanding • Anticipating
Decision-making	• Identifying options • Balancing risks and selecting option • Re-evaluation

Source: Adapted from Fletcher et al. (2003).

EXAMPLE 8.5   SCRUB PRACTITIONERS' LIST OF INTRAOPERATIVE NONTECHNICAL SKILLS (SPLINTS)

Category	Element
Situation awareness	• Gathering information • Recognising and understanding • Anticipating
Communication and teamwork	• Acting assertively • Exchanging information • Co-ordinating with others
Task management	• Planning and preparing management • Providing and maintaining standards • Coping with pressure

Source: Adapted from Mitchell et al. (2013).

skills, there is a need to train the assessors to use the behavioural marker system in advance. The effectiveness of assessor training has been reported to be mixed, but evidence suggests that improvements can be made over time (Russ et al., 2012).

ASSESSING SIMULATION EDUCATORS

It is not only important to consider the assessment of learners, but we should also consider the assessment of those delivering SBE, with the goal of providing feedback for improvement. In Chapter 3, Kirkpatrick's (1998) model of training evaluation was used to identify approaches to assessing the effectiveness of an instructional programme. There are aspects of these programmatic assessments that are relevant to simulation educators. For example, reactions questionnaires usually have items that are concerned with evaluating the performance of the person who delivered the SBE. Similarly, the OSAD and the DASH, reviewed in Chapter 7, can also be used to assess simulation educators.

It is also important to consider the performance of the learner group in any formative or summative assessments. Reviewing the performance of a learner group as a whole allows for an assessment of whether there are specific parts of the curriculum that need to be reviewed and changed, or whether there are aspects of the delivery of the education that require consideration. Also, as with learners, the feedback to educators from any assessments must be constructive and consider the psychological safety of the educator (see Chapter 6).

CONCLUSION

Assessment is an integral part of education. However, there is a need to move away from a small number of high-stakes assessments to more frequent lower-stakes formative and summative assessments. This will encourage life-long learning as opposed to a focus on 'learning the test'. We, as simulationists, also must become more comfortable with assessment of our own teaching to provide us with information on how to improve the quality of our instruction.

FURTHER READING

Gormley, G. (2011). Summative OSCEs in undergraduate medical education. *Ulster Medical Journal*, *80*(3), 127–132.

Khan, K. Z., Gaunt, K., Ramachandran, S., Pushkar, P. (2013a). The objective structured clinical examination (OSCE), AMEE guide no. 81. Part II, organisation and administration. *Medical Teacher*, *35*(9), e1447–e1463.

Khan, K. Z., Ramachandran, S., Gaunt, K., Pushkar, P. (2013b). The objective structured clinical examination (OSCE), AMEE guide no. 81. Part I, an historical and theoretical perspective. *Medical Teacher*, *35*(9), e1437–e1446.

Van Der Vleuten, C. P., Schuwirth, L. W. (2005). Assessing professional competence, from methods to programmes. *Medical Education*, *39*(3), 309–317.

ONLINE RESOURCES

- The Applied Psychology and Human Factors Group at Aberdeen University have developed a range of behavioural markers systems for healthcare and other industries. See: research.abdn.ac.uk/applied-psych-hf/non-technical-skills/
- The Observational Structured Assessment of Debriefing have a similar range of systems www.imperial.ac.uk/patient-safety-translational-research-centre/education/training-materials-for-use-in-research-and-clinical-practice/the-observational-structured/

REFERENCES

Biggs, J. (2003). Aligning teaching for constructing learning. *Higher Education Academy*, *1*(4), 1–4.

Brown, S., Pickford, R. (2006). *Assessing Skills and Practice*. Milton Park, UK: Routledge.

Chang, O. H., King, L. P., Modest, A. M., Hur, H.-C. (2016). Developing an objective structured assessment of technical skills for laparoscopic suturing and intracorporeal knot tying. *Journal of Surgical Education*, *73*(2), 258–263.

Dietz, A. S., Pronovost, P. J., Benson, K. N., Mendez-Tellez, P. A., Dwyer, C., Wyskiel, R., Rosen, M. A. (2014). A systematic review of behavioural marker systems in healthcare, what do we know about their attributes, validity and application? *BMJ Quality & Safety*, *23*(12), 1031–1039.

Epstein, R. M. (2007). Assessment in medical education. *New England Journal of Medicine*, *356*(4), 387–396.

Fletcher, G., Flin, R., McGeorge, P., Glavin, R., Maran, N., Patey, R. (2003). Anaesthetists' Non-Technical Skills (ANTS), evaluation of a behavioural marker system. *British Journal of Anaesthesia*, *90*(5), 580–588.

Flin, R., Martin, L., Goeters, K.-M., Hörmann, H.-J., Amalberti, R., Valot, C., Nijhuis, H. (2018). *Development of the NOTECHS (non-technical skills) System for Assessing Pilots' CRM Skills Human Factors and Aerospace Safety* (pp. 97–119). Milton Park, UK: Routledge.

Flin, R., O'Connor, P., Crichton, M. (2008). *Safety at the Sharp End, Training Non-technical Skills*. Aldershot: UK, Ashgate Publishing.

Gormley, G. (2011). Summative OSCEs in undergraduate medical education. *The Ulster Medical Journal*, *80*(3), 127–132.

Harden, R. M., Stevenson, M., Downie, W. W., Wilson, G. (1975). Assessment of clinical competence using objective structured examination. *British Medical Journal*, *1*(5955), 447–451.

Hatala, R., Cook, D. A., Brydges, R., Hawkins, R. (2015). Constructing a validity argument for the Objective Structured Assessment of Technical Skills (OSATS), a systematic review of validity evidence. *Advances in Health Sciences Education*, *20*(5), 1149–1175.

Ilgen, J. S., Ma, I. W., Hatala, R., Cook, D. A. (2015). A systematic review of validity evidence for checklists versus global rating scales in simulation-based assessment. *Medical Education*, *49*(2), 161–173.

Khan, K. Z., Gaunt, K., Ramachandran, S., Pushkar, P. (2013a). The objective structured clinical examination (OSCE), AMEE guide no. 81. Part II, organisation & administration. *Medical Teacher*, *35*(9), e1447–e1463.

Khan, K. Z., Ramachandran, S., Gaunt, K., Pushkar, P. (2013b). The objective structured clinical examination (OSCE), AMEE guide no. 81. Part I, an historical and theoretical perspective. *Medical Teacher*, *35*(9), e1437–e1446.

Kirkpatrick, D. L. (1998). *Evaluating Training Progams*. San Francisco: Berrett-Koehler.

Martin, J., Regehr, G., Reznick, R., Macrae, H., Murnaghan, J., Hutchison, C., Brown, M. (1997). Objective structured assessment of technical skill (OSATS) for surgical residents. *British Journal of Surgery*, *84*(2), 273–278.

Miller, G. E. (1990). The assessment of clinical skills/competence/performance. *Academic Medicine*, *65*(9), S63–67.

Mitchell, L., Flin, R., Yule, S., Mitchell, J., Coutts, K., Youngson, G. (2013). Development of a behavioural marker system for scrub practitioners' non-technical skills (SPLINTS system). *Journal of Evaluation in Clinical Practice*, *19*(2), 317–323.

O'Connor, P., Long, W. M. (2011). The development of a prototype behavioral marker system for US Navy officers of the deck. *Safety Science*, *49*(10), 1381–1387.

Pell, G., Fuller, R., Homer, M., Roberts, T. (2010). How to measure the quality of the OSCE, a review of metrics–AMEE guide no. 49. *Medical Teacher*, *32*(10), 802–811.

Pell, G., Homer, M. S., Roberts, T. E. (2008). Assessor training, its effects on criterion-based assessment in a medical context. *International Journal of Research & Method in Education*, *31*(2), 143–154.

Reid-McDermott, B., O'Connor, P., Carey, C., … Byrne, D. (2022). *A Compendium of the Steps Required to Complete 13 Essential Procedural Skills*. The Irish Centre for Applied Patient Safety and Simulation. Galway, Ireland: University of Galway.

Russ, S., Hull, L., Rout, S., Vincent, C., Darzi, A., Sevdalis, N. (2012). Observational teamwork assessment for surgery, feasibility of clinical and nonclinical assessor calibration with short-term training. *Annals of Surgery*, *255*(4), 804–809.

Schuwirth, L., Van Der Vleuten, C. (2004). Merging views on assessment. *Medical Education*, *38*(12), 1208–1210.

Shumway, J. M., Harden, R. M. (2003). The assessment of learning outcomes for the competent and reflective physician. AMEE Guide No. 25. *Medical Teacher*, *25*, 569–584.

Van Der Vleuten, C. P., Schuwirth, L. W. (2005). Assessing professional competence, from methods to programmes. *Medical Education*, *39*(3), 309–317.

9 Running a Simulation Facility

KEY POINTS

- Appropriate organisational process and supports are required to underpin a programme of simulation activities delivered through a simulation facility.
- There are eight priority areas that need to be addressed in order for a simulation facility to run effectively: (1) governance structure; (2) programme management; (3) resource management; (4) personnel; (5) staff and faculty development; (6) programme assessment; (7) integrity; and (8) promoting the activities of the simulation facility.
- Strategic planning is an approach to deciding which priority areas to focus on. A strategic plan defines a facility's strategy, or direction, and supports decisions on how to allocate resources in order to pursue specific goals.

INTRODUCTION

Many of the people involved in healthcare simulation do so because they are dedicated to delivering effective and impactful education and training – not usually because of an interest in financial management and human resources. However, it is impossible to deliver effective simulation-based education (SBE) unless the organisational process and supports are in place in order to run the facility from which the training is delivered. Despite large initial financial investments, healthcare simulation facilities may fail to thrive due to a lack of consideration of the long-term sustainability of the facility, or the business or human resources aspects of running a simulation facility. Arguably, the establishment of a simulation facility may not be the greatest challenge. Rather, engaging faculty and users, and sustaining and growing simulation activities across multiple learner groups, is the greater challenge. Therefore, to be successful, it is important to manage not only the education and training aspects of simulation, but also the 'business' of running a simulation facility.

Many challenges of resources and staff are common to all simulation facilities. However, there will also be unique challenges specific to every facility; there is no 'single best answer' for exactly how to run a simulation facility. Nevertheless, it is possible to identify those priority areas that must be addressed, and to provide guidance as to how to run a sustainable facility. This chapter is relevant not only to a dedicated simulation facility or facilities, but also for simulation programmes that may occur outside of a dedicated space (e.g., a simulation programme delivered in an Emergency Department).

CHAPTER OUTLINE

This chapter will discuss the eight priority areas that need to be addressed when running a simulation facility.

DOI: 10.1201/9781003296942-9

TABLE 9.1
Simulation Facility Priority Areas

1. Governance structure	**2. Programme management**
• Leadership	• Instructional design
• Mission and vision statement	• Policies and procedures
• Steering committee	
3. Resource management	**4. Personnel**
• Financing	• Staffing
• Selecting and purchasing equipment	• Job descriptions
• Inventorying equipment	
• Storage of equipment	
• Facilities	
5. Staff and faculty development	**6. Programme assessment**
• Education, training, and qualifications	• Evaluation
• Staff accreditation or certification	• Learner feedback
	• Faculty evaluation
	• Simulation management systems
	• Facility accreditation
7. Integrity	**8. Promoting the activities of a simulation facility**
• Adoption of a code of ethics	• Local promotion
	• Website and social media
	• National and international promotional activities

SIMULATION FACILITY PRIORITY AREAS

There are eight priority areas that we believe need to be addressed in order for a simulation facility to run effectively (see Table 9.1). These priority areas are drawn from a number of sources: (1) the core standards and criteria described by the Society of Simulation in Healthcare (2016), and the Association for Simulated Practice in Healthcare (2016); (2) the strategic plans of a number of international simulation facilities; (3) our experience of establishing the Irish Centre for Applied Patient Safety and Simulation (ICAPSS) in Galway, Ireland; and (4) a report we wrote for the Irish healthcare system on delivering simulation on clinical sites (Byrne et al., 2021).

PRIORITY AREA 1: GOVERNANCE STRUCTURE

There is a need to establish an appropriate governance structure for a simulation facility. This structure should be supported by a strategic plan (discussed later in the chapter). There are three elements to consider in this first priority area.

LEADERSHIP

There should be an identified Facility Director. A designated Facility Director should: have clear roles and responsibilities delineated in a job description for the role; have sufficient time to carry out the role; have organisational influence; be identified as part of any organisational/management structure; and be accountable for the management of simulation activities. The provision of monthly or bimonthly activity reports to executive committees are part of this role.

Mission and Vision Statements

There is a need for clear vision and mission statements for a simulation facility. These statements should be prominently placed and familiar to staff and faculty. The mission statement offers a brief summary of the purpose of the simulation facility and why it exists. For example, the mission statement for the Steinberg Facility for Simulation and Interactive Learning (2015) is: "to employ simulation in a health care context, focused on the education of health care professionals, patients and the public." The vision statement captures the aspirations of the simulation facility. It is a statement of the goals of the simulation facility. To illustrate, the vision of the ICAPSS is to "transform the delivery of healthcare through evidence-based quality improvement and education".

Steering Committee

The steering committee should have representation from all stakeholders in simulation activities (e.g., facility staff, faculty, learners, the organisation (managers, healthcare workers), and public/ patient representatives). The role of the steering committee is to develop and implement the strategic plan and promote simulation activities in the members' areas of interest and expertise. The terms of reference of the steering committee should reflect the mission of the simulation facility. Tasks of the committee include setting goals and priority areas, providing a mechanism for developing new SBE activity, scaling activities, and engaging stakeholders. The steering committee should review and update the strategic plan every 3–5 years.

PRIORITY AREA 2: PROGRAMME MANAGEMENT

The simulation programme can be defined as all of the simulation activities delivered through a simulation facility. This programme might include courses that are completely delivered in the facility (e.g. a debriefing course), supporting the simulation component of a larger course (e.g. supporting the delivery of the simulation component of the training required by trainee doctors in a particular specialty), single stand-alone training activities, and research or quality improvement activities. Consideration is required to ensure the facility is adequately supported in terms of funding, resources, and personnel to sustain these activities. It is important to ensure that there are processes in place to ensure that any changes to the programme of simulation activities delivered through the facility are reviewed, and consistent with the mission of the facility. With this in mind, there are two elements to the second priority area.

Instructional Design

As discussed in detail in Chapter 3, instructional design requires a proper design process in which the educational needs of the learners are identified, training is designed to meet these needs, and an evaluation as to whether these needs have been met by the learners. The goal of instructional design is to construct a SBE activity that optimises the learning for the participants. Therefore, we recommend the application of a systematic, and standardised, approach to instructional design such as the ADDIE model (see Chapter 3).

Policies and Procedures

Robust policies and procedures are required to support the simulation activities carried out in a simulation facility. Dongilli et al. (2021) have developed a useful simulation programme policy and procedures manual template that identifies 23 different areas that need to be addressed. These areas are:

1. General information (e.g. mission and vision statement)	14. Courses
2. Administration information (e.g. organisational chart)	15. Remediation
3. Course directors and facilitators	16. Customer relations
4. Course participants	17. Travel and meeting attendance
5. Scheduling courses and rooms	18. Research
6. Tours	19. Safety and security
7. Equipment	20. Biohazardous material
8. Supplies	21. Cadaveric use
9. Scenarios	22. Standardised patients
10. Operations	23. Simulated medical equipment and supplies in clinical settings
11. Video-recording	
12. Course observation	
13. Fiscal	

PRIORITY AREA 3: RESOURCE MANAGEMENT

Processes must be in place at a simulation facility to ensure that the facilities and equipment are available, or can be readily obtained, to support the mission and vision of the facility. There are five elements for consideration in the third priority area.

FINANCING

It is obviously important that there is sufficient funding to carry out the mission of a simulation facility. There are probably few examples of simulation facilities making a profit. To ensure sufficient funds are available requires a consideration of the costs and revenue streams. Costs associated with running a simulation facility can be broadly summarised as "stuff, staff, and space" (Senvisky et al., 2022). Costs can be divided into direct costs such as the cost of building a facility, and the cost of equipment (e.g., simulators, computers, software, consumables for delivering the training). The salaries of staff directly involved in supporting a simulation programme (e.g., simulation technicians, standardised participants) is also considered a direct cost. Indirect costs are the operational overheads. These indirect costs include those associated with depreciation of facilities or equipment, simulator warranties, and equipment repair (Senvisky et al., 2022). However, regardless of whether a cost is direct or indirect it is important that these costs are understood. It is also important to have an understanding of the cost of delivering a particular course. The cost of delivering a course is discussed in Chapter 3 within the context of evaluating the return-on-investment. Maloney and Haines (2016) also provide a good discussion of costs and benefits and the cost-effectiveness of simulation.

For many simulation facilities, revenue is derived from a number of funding streams. There may be a budget provided by the organisation of which the facility is part. There may be sponsorship for particular courses (e.g., from medical device manufacturers), or through research or education grants. Some centres may charge external learners or receive funding from training bodies to provide particular training courses. Where people are charged to attend a course it is important to know how much it costs to deliver the training to ensure that the costs are being adequately covered. Additional cost consideration may include catering, printing, and awarding Continuous Professional Development (CPD) credits.

SELECTING AND PURCHASING EQUIPMENT

The capital cost of purchasing equipment is often the main consideration. However, there is also a need to consider the durability, cost of replacement parts, compatibility and ease of storage of any equipment. This information can be gathered by talking to the manufacturer and using the equipment yourself. It is also important to talk to people who have actually purchased and have experience in using a piece of equipment for teaching. The most important consideration is to align what skill you intend to teach with the simulator you choose. This 'functional-task alignment' moves the conversation away from the 'fidelity' of the simulator to the more practical functionality of the product. Another important consideration when selecting equipment is the learner population who will be using the equipment. To illustrate, it is unlikely to be necessary to purchase a highly sophisticated manikin for use by medical students. If the facility is part of a larger organisation, such as a hospital or university, there are likely to be procurement processes and rules that have to be followed for transparency and to achieve best value (e.g., obtaining three quotes for purchases or running a mini-competition between vendors above a certain cost threshold). Additional costs, such as tax, import duties, and shipping costs, can increase the listed cost of simulators. It is important that the person responsible for purchasing at the facility is both familiar with, and follows, these processes.

Inventorying Equipment

An accurate record should be kept of the equipment that has been purchased for the facility. There should be an inventory of the equipment that includes: date of purchase, duration of warranty, the replacement parts required, and the specifications of the simulation equipment.

Storage of Equipment

Space for storage of equipment at a simulation facility is often limited. It is suggested that the ideal minimum storage space requirement is a quarter of the floor space. However, we appreciate that this is often not possible. Storage type and design should be considered in the context of the activities in the facility. For example, cold storage and storage for specialist waste disposal may be required if animal parts are being prepared or used for surgical skills training, roller storage may be required for larger simulators. Heavy simulators cannot be stored at height for health and safety reasons and a hoist may be required for moving heavy adult manikins.

Facilities

Most simulation facilities are retrofitted and are not purpose-built, and often simulation staff do the best with what is available. Nevertheless, should funding become available to improve the facilities, it is important that the money is spent effectively. Potential improvements may include: sound proofing, use of piped gases, consideration of adjacencies for noise control, one-way mirrors and lighting, room configuration, flexible and mobile furniture, improved storage, and audio-visual or learning management systems. It is very useful to visit other simulation facilities and talk to staff about what they did, and, more importantly, to hear what they would do differently. It is also useful to obtain advice from architects and builders who have developed clinical spaces – particularly when it comes to replicating these spaces in the simulation facility and understanding the limitations as well as the health and safety challenges.

PRIORITY AREA 4: PERSONNEL

People are critical to the success of the facility. This includes the facility staff, faculty, and simulation management team. This fourth priority area has two elements.

STAFFING

The number of staff required in a simulation facility depends on the volume of activities, the number of courses, and the type of activities (e.g., undergraduate, postgraduate, or external teaching, quality improvement, research, systems testing or analysis). The staff can be broadly divided into core simulation staff and simulation faculty. Core staff include simulation technicians, administrative support, academic staff (e.g., lecturers in simulation, psychology), simulation educators (clinical staff) and the directors of simulation and research. The learning activities are usually supported by faculty who lead or support the design, delivery and debrief of a simulation course. These include clinical staff who are interested in SBE and who support the delivery of curricular content for an undergraduate medical or nursing school or for a postgraduate training body. Faculty also include hospital staff who are using simulation for quality improvement purposes or to examine particular processes and systems. The development needs of core staff and faculty differ. Core staff require a broad understanding of the requirements for running a simulation facility in order to support the activities. Faculty require support to develop skills in simulation design and debriefing in their specialist area.

JOB DESCRIPTIONS

Job descriptions should be developed for specific simulation roles, such as: Facility Director, standardised patient educators, technical staff, facility managers, and administrative staff. Roche et al. (2022) identified the large range of competencies required of a simulation technician, and found there is considerable variability in the desired competencies across different simulation technician job adverts. Consideration should also be given to how these positions align with the pay scales of the larger organisation in which the simulation facility is situated.

PRIORITY AREA 5: FACULTY AND STAFF DEVELOPMENT

Although this is beginning to change, there is no specific career path or training pipeline for simulation educators, simulation technicians, or administrative staff. By way of illustration, at our simulation facility we have people with a clinical background, but also staff with experience in medical science, the military, farming, information technology, and the beauty industry. Therefore, it is important to consider how staff from a range of very different backgrounds should be trained and developed.

EDUCATION, TRAINING, AND QUALIFICATIONS

It is important that simulation faculty and core staff are provided with education and training opportunities in order to support their professional development. This is particularly important for those faculty who do not have a background in simulation. There are an increasing number of simulation-based graduate programmes (e.g., the Diploma and Masters in Healthcare Simulation and Patient Safety at the University of Galway). Core simulation staff should have a qualification and/or be accredited with a simulation accrediting body (discussed below). For faculty, it is not essential to have a postgraduate qualification in simulation – provided they have an understanding of SBE, instructional design and delivery and they are supported by core simulation staff. One approach to begin building faculty expertise is to facilitate the observation, participation, and support of existing simulation activities. As the faculty become more experienced, they can gradually become involved in debriefing and assessment activities. Short courses (e.g. train-the-trainer, debriefing) are particularly useful to help faculty rapidly build knowledge and expertise. Such training is available at many simulation facilities and offered by a number of simulation societies.

Core staff such as simulation technicians require training in specific technical areas in order to perform their role effectively (e.g., audio-visual, online learning, simulated participant education, simulator maintenance). Short courses in the more technical aspects of simulation are available from simulation societies and associations (see the online resources at the end of this chapter for some examples). Healthcare simulation societies generally hold workshops before or during the annual conference and simulation manufacturing companies often support or provide training and workshops. There are several simulation technician international groups and simulation societies also have special interest groups for technical staff. Simulation facilities should hold annual training and train the trainer workshops for staff and faculty and host journal clubs to develop a community of simulation practice in their organisations. It is also recommended that staff and faculty are supported to visit, and build networks, with technicians from other facilities in order to share expertise and knowledge.

STAFF ACCREDITATION OR CERTIFICATION

Simulation staff accreditation or certification is valuable because it demonstrates that a level of competence has been achieved in the delivery of simulation. It is particularly important for simulation facilities to support core staff in becoming accredited. Seeking accreditation is helpful for staff as it provides guidance on the areas in which competency is required. Simulation societies offer different levels of certification and accreditation based on experience and level of leadership in simulation activities. In addition, achieving accreditation demonstrates to the learners, and members of the wider organisation, that the staff in the facility are competent to deliver SBE and training. Individual accreditation can be sought from the Association for Simulated Practice in Healthcare (ASPiH) and the Society for Simulation in Europe (SESAM), for educators. Certification for educators and simulation technicians can be obtained through the Society for Simulation in Healthcare (SSH).

PRIORITY AREA 6: PROGRAMME ASSESSMENT

It is important that there are procedures and processes in place to assess the quality of the activities delivered in a simulation programme. This priority area has five elements.

EVALUATION

Evaluation is particularly important for new SBE activities. Evaluation of programmes is discussed in detail in Chapter 3 on instructional design. However, it is also necessary to evaluate existing SBE activities to ensure they are still achieving the learning outcomes, and identify whether any updates or changes are required. The ADDIE model (discussed in Chapter 3) can provide a framework for changing an existing SBE activity based upon feedback from evaluation.

LEARNER FEEDBACK

Participant feedback following the completion of a simulation activity should be collected regularly in order to assess the reactions of the learners. This can be achieved using online or paper-based surveys circulated at the end of an education activity (see the evaluation section of Chapter 3). Rather than only relying on Likert-scale responses, free text response questions can be used in order to elicit suggestions on how the SBE activity can be improved and how the learning from simulation can be applied, or be made more relevant, to clinical practice.

FACULTY EVALUATION

Periodic formative evaluation of the faculty is important to assess how the faculty are delivering the training, and to give feedback to them on what they are doing well and where improvements could be made. Debriefing assessment tools for faulty have been developed and are discussed in detail in Chapter 7 of this book.

SIMULATION MANAGEMENT SYSTEMS

There are simulation management systems (SMS) available that support audio-visual requirements, running a facility, and learning activity management. These systems can be configured so that the details of simulation events or courses of instruction can be stored in detail, and learner feedback can be collated.

FACILITY ACCREDITATION

In addition to accreditation of simulation facility staff, it is also worth considering obtaining accreditation for the simulation facility. Accreditation involves measuring the activities of the facility against a set of standards. Accreditation demonstrates to learners, and the larger organisation, that simulation activities have been benchmarked against best practice. The accreditation process involves the submission of evidence of excellence in SBE. The collation of the evidence is a useful self-assessment process to undertake. Following submission of the evidence, an inspection of the facility follows and includes interviews with stakeholders, staff and learners. Facility accreditation can be sought from simulation societies, such as ASPiH, SSH, SESAM, or the Network of Accredited Skills Centres in Europe (NASCE).

PRIORITY AREA 7: INTEGRITY

It is important that staff working at a simulation facility are aware of, and follow, the ethical standards in the delivery of education and training, as well as any other activities carried out by the facility (e.g., research).

ADOPTION OF A CODE OF ETHICS

The Society for Simulation in Healthcare (SSH; 2018) has developed a code of ethics for healthcare simulationists. The SSH code of ethics identifies six key aspirational values important to the practice of simulation: (1) integrity (display honesty, truthfulness, fairness, and good judgement); (2) transparency (display clarity in the design, communication, and decision-making processes in simulation activities); (3) mutual respect (respect the rights, dignity, and worth of all); (4) professionalism (uphold the professional standards inherent in healthcare simulation); (5) accountability (facility staff are accountable for their decisions and actions); and (6) results orientation (support activities that enhance the quality of the profession and healthcare systems). This code of ethics should be aligned with those of the wider organisation of which the simulation facility is part. It is also important to be aware of, and practice, ethical conduct in any research undertaken at the facility (see Chapter 10) and quality improvement projects (see Chapter 11).

PRIORITY AREA 8: PROMOTING THE ACTIVITIES OF A SIMULATION FACILITY

It is important that the activities of the simulation facility are recorded, made available to stakeholders (management, funders, accrediting bodies), and promoted. This is particularly the case for a new facility, or where there has been a change in the vision or mission of a facility. Record keeping forms a critical part of promotion and many other priority areas such as governance, resource management, and accreditation. This final priority area has three elements.

LOCAL PROMOTION

It is important to demonstrate how the facility can support the delivery of education and training, as well as the wider needs of organisations such as research and quality improvement activities locally. The Facility Director should give regular updates to the senior management of any wider organisation or stakeholder group of which the facility is part. It is also important to inform members of the wider organisation what the facility has done, and what it can do to support teaching, research, and quality improvement activities. This can be achieved through engagement with relevant healthcare and university executives and management committees and through presentations (e.g., Grand Rounds). Organising presentations and tours of the facility for visitors and for simulated patients is a good way to encourage patient and community interest in simulation activities which may lead to future participation in simulation activities or patient and public involvement (PPI) groups.

WEBSITE AND SOCIAL MEDIA

A website or webpage that displays the facility's mission and vision and code of ethics should be developed. This website should include details of key staff members, equipment available, and educational and research activities. It is also recommended that social media is used to promote training and other activities carried out in the facility.

NATIONAL AND INTERNATIONAL PROMOTIONAL ACTIVITIES

Having a website and active social media feed are useful for the national and international promotion of the facility and its activities. However, staff and faculty should develop national and international recognition through the delivery of presentations and workshops at simulation conferences, publications in simulation journals, or achieving accreditation from a simulation society (see the links to these societies at the end of this chapter).

SIMULATION FACILITY STRATEGIC PLANNING

A recommended approach to deciding which priority areas to focus upon is through strategic planning. A strategic plan defines the strategy, or direction, and supports decisions on how to allocate resources in order to pursue specific goals. Strategic plans usually cover time periods measured in years rather than months. For example, a 3-to-5-year plan would be appropriate for larger goals. The importance for a simulation facility to have a strategic plan is recognised by both the Society for Simulation in Healthcare and the Association for Simulated Practice in Healthcare.

Although the strategic planning process can be led by the Facility Director, it is ultimately a team effort that is coordinated by the steering committee with representation from all stakeholders. The planning process is as important as the delivery of the plan as it generates a collaborative spirit. Table 9.2 provides an overview of a 'classic' approach to strategic planning in five stages. While it is listed as a series of linear steps, it is often much more complex as simulation activities are often running at the same time as planning is happening. An important consideration in getting the strategic plan implemented is achieving buy-in from internal and external stakeholders. This requires the building of relationships and support from the change management that includes internal and external advocacy and the building of relationships with stakeholders. For a detailed outline of strategic planning for a simulation facility, we recommend reading the paper by O'Connor et al. (2023).

TABLE 9.2

Summary of Stages in the Development of a Strategic Plan

Stage 1. Define the mission, vision and values – the guiding forces behind facilities strategic planning and performance assessment activities.

- *1A. Mission statement* – describes the purpose of the simulation facility.
- *1B. Vision* – what the facility hopes to be achieve following the implementation of the strategic plan.
- *1C. Values* – the core beliefs of those affiliated with the centre.

Stage 2: Strategic formulation – the formation of a strategy to meet the mission, vision, and values of the facility.

- *2A. Analysing the external environment* – identifying any external factors that can impact the facility (e.g., learners, suppliers).
- *2B. Analysing the internal environment* identifying any internal factors that can impact the facility (e.g., technical personnel, training courses).
- *2C. SWOT analysis* – completion of a Strengths, Weakness, Opportunities, and Threats (SWOT) analysis to identify all potential actions that could be completed.
- *2D. Strategic alternatives* – collation of potential actions from the SWOT analysis.
- *2E. Strategic areas and objectives* – identify a limited number of strategic areas to focus on.

Stage 3: Operational planning – ensures that each strategic objective is specific, practical, and recognisable.

Stage 4: Assessing the results – the steering committee must retain oversight of whether specific objectives are being achieved.

Stage 5: Reformulating the strategy – the steering committee must retain oversight of the strategy and consider making changes if there are issues with meeting any of the stated objectives.

CONCLUSIONS

To achieve success and growth in activities, a simulation facility must be sustainable, and have the resources required to deliver on the mission of the facility. This requires effective running of the 'business' side of a simulation facility. The seven priority areas are all important to establishing and maintaining the activities of a simulation facility. However, they do not all need to be addressed at once. Developing a strategic plan, with input from a range of stakeholders, will provide direction on which priority area (or areas) should be focused upon in the short to medium term, and ensure that the core business of delivering simulation activities is not negatively impacted.

FURTHER READING

Byrne. D., O'Dowd, E., Lydon, S., Reid McDermott, B., O'Connor, P. (2021). *The National Simulation Strategic Guide for the Implementation of Simulation on Clinical Sites*. Galway, Ireland: University of Galway. DOI: 10.13025/cn0z-bp50.

Dongilli. T., Gavilanes, J., Shekhter, I., Kuki, A., Wong, J., Howard, V., Hara, K., Lin, M. (2021). *SSH Simulation Program Policy and Procedure Manual Model Template*. Minneapolis, MN: Society for Simulation in Healthcare.

Maloney, S., Haines, T. (2016). Issues of cost-benefit and cost-effectiveness for simulation in health professions education. *Advances in Simulation*, 1, 13.

O'Connor, P., O'Dowd, E., Lydon, S., Byrne, D. (2023). Developing a strategic plan for a healthcare simulation facility. *International Journal of Healthcare Simulation*. DOI: 10.54531/gcih5434.

Roche, A., Condron, C. Eppich, W., O'Connor, P. (2023). A mixed methods study identifying the competencies of healthcare simulation technicians. *Simulation in Healthcare*. DOI: 10.1097/SIH.0000000000000682.

Senvisky, J.M., McKenna, R.T., Okuda, Y. (2022). *Financing and Funding a Simulation Center*. In: StatPearls [Internet]. Treasure Island, Florida: StatPearls Publishing.

Society of Simulation in Healthcare Code of Ethics Working Group (2018). *Healthcare Simulationists Code of Ethics*. Available from: www.ssih.org/SSH-Resources/Code-of-Ethics

Watts, P. I., Rossler, K., Bowler, F., Miller, C., Charnetski, M., Decker, S., … Hallmark, B. (2021). Onward and upward: Introducing the healthcare simulation standards of best practice. *Clinical Simulation in Nursing*, *58*, 1–4.

ONLINE RESOURCES

- Examples of simulation policies and procedure manuals: www.healthysimulation. com/33051/clinical-simulation-policies-procedures/

ACCREDITATION

- Association for Simulated Practice in Healthcare: aspih.org.uk/accreditation/
- Society for Simulation in Europe: www.sesam-web.org/accreditation
- Society for Simulation in Healthcare: www.ssih.org/Credentialing/Accreditation
- Network of Accredited Skills Centres in Europe: nascenet.org

EXAMPLES OF ORGANISATIONS WHO DELIVER SHORT COURSES IN SIMULATION

- Scottish Centre for Simulation & Clinical Human Factors courses: scschf.org/courses/
- Dundee Institute of Healthcare Simulation (DIHS): dihs.dundee.ac.uk
- Centre for Medical Simulation Instructor Training: harvardmedsim.org/training/ simulation-instructor-training/
- Great Ormond Street Hospital for Children Debriefing course: www.gosh.nhs.uk/ working-here/gosh-learning-academy/clinical-simulation-centre/simulation-courses/
- Royal College of Physicians UK 'Getting the most out of simulation: debriefing and scenario writing in simulation': www.rcplondon.ac.uk/education-practice/courses/ getting-most-out-simulation-debriefing-and-screnario-writing-simulation

OTHER ONLINE RESOURCES

- The website www.healthysimulation.com provides links to upcoming courses.
- The Society for Simulation in Healthcare (SSH) has a live learning centre which offers various courses relating to simulation, ranging from debriefing and scenario development to 3D printing and the use of virtual reality: https://www.ssih.org/Professional-Development/ Online-Learning/Live-Learning-Center
- SimGHOST is an organisation with resources on simulation with a simulation technician focus: simghosts.org

REFERENCES

Association for Simulated Practice in Healthcare. (2016). Simulation-Based Education in Healthcare- Standards Framework and Guidance.

Byrne, D., O'Dowd, E., Lydon, S., Reid McDermott, B., O'Connor, P. (2021). *The National Simulation Strategic Guide for the Implementation of Simulation on Clinical Sites*. Galway, Ireland: University of Galway.

Dongilli, T., Gavilanes, J., Shekhter, I., Kuki, A., Wong, J., Howard, V., Hara, K., Lin, M. (2021). *SSH Simulation Program Policy and Procedure Manual Model Template*. Minneapolis, MN: Society for Simulation in Healthcare.

Maloney, S., Haines, T. (2016). Issues of cost–benefit and cost-effectiveness for simulation in health professions education. *Advances in Simulation*, *1*(1), 13.

O'Connor, P., O'Dowd, E., Lydon, S., Byrne, D. (2023). Developing a strategic plan for a healthcare simulation facility. *International Journal of Healthcare Simulation*. DOI: 10.54531/gcih5434.

Roche, A. F., Condron, C. M., Eppich, W. J., O'Connor, P. E. (2022). A mixed methods study identifying the competencies of healthcare simulation technicians. *Simulation in Healthcare*. DOI: 10.1097/SIH.0000000000000682.

Senvisky, J. M., McKenna, R. T., Okuda, Y. (2022). *Financing and Funding a Simulation Center*. Treasure Island, FL: StatPearls Publishing.

Society for Simulation in Healthcare. (2016). Committee for Accreditation of Healthcare Simulation Programs: CORE Standards and Measurement Criteria.

Society of Simulation in Healthcare Code of Ethics Working Group. (2018). Healthcare Simultionists Code of Ethics. http://www.ssih.org/SSH-Resources/Code-of-Ethics

Steinberg Centre for Simulation and Interactive Learning McGill University. (2015). The Steinberg Centre for Simulation and Interactive: A Forward View.

10 Using Simulation for Research

KEY POINTS

- Research *about* simulation: answers research questions in which the focus is on simulation itself (e.g., evaluating the efficacy of simulation-based education).
- Research *through* simulation: the focus of this research is not simulation itself, but rather the uses of simulation as a method/tool for research (e.g., evaluating the effectiveness of different alarm frequencies).
- Research must be guided by a good research question.
- Research should be feasible, interesting, novel, ethical, and relevant.
- There are many different outlets to publish and share simulation research.

INTRODUCTION

As the use of simulation has become more common in healthcare education, there has been an exponential rise in the number of research articles published and a corresponding increase in the outlets that publish this research (Walsh et al., 2018). However, simulation research is not equally distributed across the world's simulation centres. In a survey of 42 simulation centres from across the world, only 26 (62%) reported research activities related to simulation. Moreover, of the research publications reported, 98% originate from just six centres (Qayumi et al., 2014). Therefore, the goal of this chapter is to encourage simulation research, and to broaden the number of centres, and individuals, contributing to the academic literature and presenting at conferences.

CHAPTER OVERVIEW

This chapter will:

- introduce different types of simulation research;
- provide guidance on developing a research question and how to carry out simulation research;
- provide guidance on writing a simulation research publication; and
- provide some thoughts on how to decide where to present or publish simulation research.

TYPES OF SIMULATION RESEARCH

There are two broad categories of simulation research:

- research *about* simulation: this type of research answers the research questions in which the focus is on simulation itself (e.g., evaluating the efficacy of a simulation-based training – see Chapter 3); and
- research *through* simulation: the focus of this research is not simulation itself, but rather uses simulation as a method/tool for research (e.g., evaluating the effectiveness of different alarm frequencies in a simulated clinical environment Lamé & Dixon-Woods, 2020)

DOI: 10.1201/9781003296942-10

RESEARCH ABOUT SIMULATION

Research about simulation dominates the area of healthcare simulation research (O'Connor, 2020; Walsh et al., 2018). A bibliometric review of the 100 most cited articles in healthcare simulation found that the majority of studies (86%) were concerned with education and training; of those, 28% were concerned with evaluating the impact of simulation-based interventions (Walsh et al., 2018). Similarly, the research priorities identified by simulation societies/organisations also focus on research about simulation. To illustrate, the top research questions identified by simulation experts in a study by the Simulation in Healthcare Research Committee were concerned with:

1. the impact of system-level simulation interventions on system efficiency, patient safety, and patient outcomes;
2. the return on investment of simulation for healthcare systems; and
3. whether a dose–response relationship exists between simulation training and performance/ patient outcomes.

(Anton et al., 2022)

As a result of the large volume of research about simulation, there is now sufficient evidence that healthcare simulation is an effective educational intervention (McGaghie et al., 2010; Walsh et al., 2018). Therefore, future research about simulation must shift the focus from questions of "Does healthcare simulation work?" to the more nuanced issues, such as the impact of the ratio of clinical hours to simulation time (see Example 10.1).

EXAMPLE 10.1   NATIONAL COUNCIL OF STATE BOARDS OF NURSING SIMULATION STUDY

This paper describes a longitudinal, randomised, controlled trial to assess the impact of replacing clinical hours with simulation in nursing education (Hayden et al., 2014). A total of 666 nursing students from 10 US programmes were randomised into one of three groups:

1. **Control**: Students who had traditional clinical experiences.
2. **25% group**: Students who had 25% of traditional clinical hours replaced by simulation.
3. **50% group**: Students who had 50% of traditional clinical hours replaced by simulation.

At the end of the nursing programme, there were no statistically significant differences in clinical competency, nursing knowledge, or licensing exam pass rate across the three groups. The study cohort was also followed for the first six months of clinical practice. There were no differences in ratings of overall clinical competency and readiness for practice. The results of this study provide evidence that substituting clinical hours with simulation for up to half of traditional clinical hours does not have an impact on educational outcomes.

RESEARCH THROUGH SIMULATION

In healthcare, research through simulation is considerably less common than research about simulation (see Example 10.2 for an example of research through simulation). This is the opposite to other industries in which research through simulation dominates. To illustrate, flight simulators have been used to answer a range of research questions including: what is the impact of workload on pilot performance? (Gabriel et al., 2016); what is the effect of pilot fatigue on

EXAMPLE 10.2   THE QUALITY OF CHEST COMPRESSIONS DELIVERED IN A SIMULATED AMBULANCE

A randomised, counterbalanced study was carried out with 24 paramedic students in order to assess the efficacy of chest compressions while seated versus standing (Mullin et al., 2020). Simulated chest compressions were performed in a stationary ambulance on a cardiopulmonary resuscitation (CPR) manikin for two minutes from either an unsecured standing position or a secured and seated position.

The mean total number of chest compressions, and the compression rate, was not significantly different when delivered from the two positions. However, chest compressions performed in the unsecured standing position yielded a significantly greater mean depth (52 mm) than when performed in the seated secured position (26 mm). Moreover, the standing unsecured position produced a significantly higher percentage (83%) of correct compressions, as compared to the seated secured position. It was concluded that there is a need to consider how training, technologies, and ambulance design can impact the quality of chest compressions without the need to compromise the safety of the paramedic delivering patient care (Mullin et al., 2020).

performance? (Morris & Miller, 1996); and how do pilots react to flight deck alerts? (Zheng et al., 2014). Therefore, in agreement with other authors, we believe the potential to utilise simulation for conducting research in healthcare is under-exploited (Lamé & Dixon-Woods, 2020).

CONDUCTING SIMULATION RESEARCH

You may get a research idea from reading a paper, attending a conference, talking to colleagues, or from your own experience. A good research question should be appropriate, meaningful, and purposeful (Stone, 2002). A study must be guided by a good research question. The FINER (feasible, interesting, novel, ethical, and relevant; Hulley et al., 2009) criteria is a useful approach to developing your research idea into a research question.

- *Is the research feasible?* You need to consider whether the research you want to complete can be executed with the time and resources you have available. You may consider completing a small feasibility study.
- *Is the research interesting?* You need to consider whether others will be interested in the findings from your research – particularly if you intend to publish your findings (see below). Discuss your ideas with colleagues, and have a look at the research literature to see if there is any discourse or debate around your research idea.
- *Is the research novel?* Check in the literature to make sure that what you are proposing has not been done previously. It is unlikely that what you are considering will be completely new. However, unless there is good reason (e.g., unusual or unexpected findings), it is not generally recommended to completely replicate an existing study.
- *Is the research ethical?* You need to ensure that your proposed research is ethical and that you have considered, and minimised, any potential harm and/or risks to the participants. You also must ensure that the participants have consented to participate in your research study. Before you start recruiting participants, you must have obtained approval for your research from a relevant ethics board. You should not underestimate the time this can take, and should factor this into your research plan.
- *Is the research relevant?* You need to consider the relevance of what you are planning is for the wider simulation community. You want your research to have an impact on knowledge

or practice. The potential relevance can be established by a review of the literature, and talking to colleagues and other simulationists about your plan. If the impact of your research only matters locally, it may be that that it is not worth the effort to complete.

Once you have decided on an appropriate research question, you then need to decide how you will answer it. The broadest categorisation of research designs is either positivist or interpretive (Bhattacherjee, 2012). Positivist research designs are generally concerned with testing hypotheses, and involve the collection of numerical or quantitative data. Examples of positivist designs include experimental (or quasi-experimental) studies, or survey research that utilises numerical scales in order to carry out statistical tests. In contrast, interpretivist research is focused on understanding a phenomenon based upon the subjective experiences of individuals. Common interpretivist methodologies are interviews and observations. These interview transcripts or observation notes are then analysed using approaches such as thematic analysis in order to understand the phenomenon of interest. Increasingly, researchers are carrying out mixed methods research that combines positivist and interpretive approaches.

Neither of these approaches to research is better or easier than the other. The approach you take often depends on your question and the type of information that your question calls for; this may depend on how your question is phrased. For example, you may wish to understand learner stress when engaged in a trauma simulation. A question such as 'how do junior doctors respond to stress in a simulated trauma event?' could be answered by taking a positivist approach by measuring cortisol levels, heart rate, galvanic skin response, etc. Alternatively, you could take an interpretive approach and ask the participants about their subjective experience of stress during the simulation and how that may have affected their performance. You could also take a mixed methods approach and do both. However, whichever approach you decide to use, it is important that you follow a rigorous, repeatable and structured approach and, if necessary, take advice from an experienced researcher. We would certainly recommend a team approach to research. It is very challenging to carry out even a small project alone.

Once you have decided on an approach, you then need to develop a research protocol, and a methodology for carrying it out. It is beyond the scope of the chapter to provide a detailed discussion on how to design and carry out simulation research – this would be a whole book in itself. There is also already a huge existing literature on conducting research. A book edited by Nestel et al. (2019) provides specific guidance on conducting healthcare simulation research. Medical education and psychology research methods textbooks may also provide useful guidance (e.g., Cleland & Durning, 2015). We recommend the psychology research methods book written by Howitt and Cramer (2020) to our students completing a Master's thesis in Healthcare Simulation and Patient Safety.

WRITING A SIMULATION RESEARCH PUBLICATION

Once you have completed your research study, you should consider how you will share the findings. Publication of simulation research is desirable from a career perspective, as well as to allow you to contribute to the knowledge base in your area or research. If you conduct research and it is not published or shared, then, as far as others know, it did not happen. As discussed above, there is a huge amount published on how to carry out research. However, there is much less literature describing how to write up and share a research project's findings. Therefore, we will provide some guidance on these tasks based upon our experience of supervising postgraduate research students, reviewing papers, editing journals, and publishing our own research studies.

When writing your manuscript, it is desirable to follow a set of reporting guidelines that are appropriate for the type of study that you have carried out. These guidelines provide a framework for what you should consider, and report, when describing your research. There are a range of published guidelines that cover almost every conceivable approach to research. The equator network (www.equator-network.org) is a very good starting point to find a set of reporting guidelines suitable for your research study. Also, Cheng et al. (2016) have developed reporting guidelines specifically for simulation research. Rather than going through all of these reporting guidelines, we will provide some generic recommendations for writing your manuscript that should be relevant regardless of the approach you have taken to answer your research question.

TITLE AND ABSTRACT

The title and abstract of your paper are extremely important, although they can sometimes be treated as a bit of an after-thought by the researcher. The reason they are so crucial is that the title and abstract are the first, and possibly only, part of the paper that someone will read. The title should provide some indication of the study's design and contain commonly used terms. To illustrate, the title of the Example 10.1 paper is: "*A longitudinal, randomised, controlled study replacing clinical hours with simulation in prelicensure nursing education*". The title of the Example 10.2 paper is: "*The effect of operator position on the quality of chest compressions delivered in a simulated ambulance*."

The abstract should be a short (generally 200–250 words) stand-alone summary of your paper. Oftentimes, journals will require a particular structure for the abstract. A common structure required by journals is: background, objectives, method, results, and conclusions. It is recommended that the abstract should be the final part of the paper that is written.

INTRODUCTION

The introduction should provide an overview of the background and rationale for your research. The introduction should start broadly, and then become more focused on the specific purpose of the study. To illustrate, the introduction to the study in Example 10.1 opens with:

> Nursing education in the United States is at the crossroads of tradition and innovation. High-fidelity simulation is emerging to address 21st-century clinical education needs and move nursing forward into a new era of learning and critical thinking.
>
> *(Hayden et al., 2014: S4)*

This introduction then closes with:

> The NCSBN National Simulation Study, a longitudinal, randomised, controlled trial using nursing programmes across the United States, is the largest, most comprehensive study to date that explores whether simulated clinical experiences can be substituted effectively for traditional clinical experiences in the undergraduate nursing programme.
>
> *(Hayden et al., 2014: S4)*

Similarly, for the study described in Example 10.2, the introduction begins with:

> Ambulances are clinical environments in which patient care is initiated or maintained, but this setting poses safety risks for paramedics during transport.
>
> *(Mullin et al., 2020: 55)*

This introduction then ends with:

> There is a dearth of research that directly compares the quality of chest compressions delivered in an ambulance setting between a standing and unsecured position and a seated and secured position. This data is important for considering how to deliver optimum care to patients in an ambulance while preserving the safety of the paramedic.
>
> *(Mullin et al., 2020: 56)*

The final part of the introduction should then finish with the aims of the study. Stating the aims is important and there should be a clear and concise explanation of what the study aims to find out. The aims of the study described in Example 10.1 are:

To provide Boards of Nursing with evidence on nursing knowledge, clinical competency, and the transferability of learning from the simulation laboratory to the clinical setting.

(Hayden et al., 2014: S6)

For Example 10.2 the aim is to examine:

The effectiveness of chest compressions from two conditions will be compared during simulated resuscitation in a stationary ambulance: from a standing unsecured position, or from a seated and secured position.

(Mullin et al., 2020: 56)

When writing the introduction, it is important to avoid explaining how the study was carried out (save this for the Method section), or speculating too much about what you found (save this for the Results section). Finally, make sure that any assertions made are supported by appropriate references.

METHOD

This is the section where you explain what you did in the study. Consider this to be a 'recipe' for how the study was carried out. You should provide a sufficient amount of information that would allow someone to replicate what was done. Typical headings for the methodology section of a research study are:

- *Context/setting* – What is the background to where/or with whom you did the research? (e.g., interns in a large teaching hospital in the west of Ireland).
- *Design* – What research design did you use? (e.g., randomised controlled design, qualitative interviews).
- *Ethical approval* – What is the name of the ethics board that provided ethical approval for your research, and what is the reference number of the approval?
- *Recruitment* – How did you recruit participants? (e.g., word of mouth, email).
- *Participants* – Who are the participants in your research? (e.g., Emergency Medicine staff).
- *Materials* – What materials/equipment did you use to carry out your research? (e.g., a specific type of simulator, interview protocol).
- *Procedure* – How was the data collected? This section is a chronological description of exactly how the data was collected.
- *Analysis* – What type of analysis was carried out? (e.g., statistical tests, approaches to analysing qualitative data such as thematic analysis).

RESULTS

This is the section where you describe the findings from your study. Make sure that your results provide the answer to the research question that you stated in the introduction. Your results should be easy to follow and laid out using appropriate headings/subheadings. Give careful consideration as to how you present the results, and whether they would be more clearly presented in text, table, or as a figure. Take care with presenting your results twice (e.g., do not present the same information in text and a table). Also, do not discuss your findings in the results section- just present the results.

DISCUSSION

In our experience of student supervision, writing papers, and reviewing journal articles, it is clear that the discussion is the hardest part of a research paper to write – no matter how experienced you are as a researcher. Arguably, the discussion is the most important section of a paper and the part that people are most likely to read (after the abstract). This is the section of the paper where you interpret the findings of your research. Just like the other parts of a research paper, there is a standard format for how to structure your discussion.

Good advice is to start the discussion with a short, pithy summary of the main findings of the study – this should be linked back to the stated objectives of the study. In this first paragraph you are really reminding the reader of the purpose of the study.

> Delivering effective chest compressions during a cardiopulmonary arrest is crucial…The study reported in this paper is one of a few studies that have specifically examined the impact of body position of the paramedic on the quality of chest compressions, and was the only study of which the authors are aware of that compares standing versus seated positions… These findings have implications for the training of paramedics to deliver chest compressions, ambulance design, and the use of technologies such as mechanical CPR devices and real-time feedback.
>
> *(Mullin et al., 2020: 59)*

Following the opening paragraph, you should then address the following points:

- comment on the implications of the findings of the study;
- address the research question(s) you delineated in the introduction;
- compare and contrast your findings with any other relevant work in the field;
- outline the strengths and limitations of the study; and
- end with a reflection on ideas for future research and recommendations for practice.

Referencing. It is important to use the referencing style of your chosen journal. Many journals also have guidance on the number of references that you can use, so make sure you do not exceed the maximum allowed. Give careful consideration to how you reference. Avoid more than one or two direct quotes at a maximum in your manuscript. Also, ensure that you are providing appropriate references to back up any points you are making in your manuscript.

AUTHORSHIP

Authorship has the potential to be contentious and lead to arguments within a research project team. The first decision to be made on authorship is who should be listed as an author. The International Committee of Medical Journal Editors (2021) has identified four criteria for authorship. A potential author must have:

1. made substantial contributions to the conception or design of the work; or the acquisition, analysis, or interpretation of data for the work; AND
2. drafted the work or revised it critically for important intellectual content; AND
3. provided final approval of the of the work to be published; AND
4. agreed to be accountable for all aspects of the work and ensure that questions related to the accuracy or integrity of any part of the work are appropriately investigated and resolved.

Once the list of authors is established, the next decision to be made is the order in which the authors should be listed on the manuscript. Riesenberg and Lundberg (1990) made the following recommendations for determining the sequence of author:

1. The first author should be that person who contributed most to the work, including the writing of the manuscript.
2. The sequence of authors should be determined by the relative overall contributions to the manuscript.

3. It is common practice, at least in healthcare, for the 'senior author' to be listed last – regardless of his or her contribution. However, it is important that the senior author, like all other authors, should meet all criteria for authorship.

The senior author may be the person who received the funding for the work, or the research group leader. Where the first author is a research student, the senior author is generally the student's supervisor. Our suggestion for avoiding arguments about authorship is to be very transparent about authorship and the responsibilities of each author from the planning stage of the work. The responsibilities and order of authorship should be discussed by the research team. As the research project progresses, it may be there are changes in the quantity of work carried out by each author, or that aspects of the work require more effort than anticipated. Therefore, it is important for there to be some flexibility in the authorship and consider how the order might change. Also, it is important for the authors themselves to be sensible and pragmatic about authorship. For example, it is unlikely to be worthwhile falling out with everyone on the research team because you think you should be fourth instead of fifth author on a paper.

CHOOSING WHERE TO PUBLISH SIMULATION RESEARCH

Identifying were to publish your research can be challenging. As listed in Chapter 1, there are a number of healthcare simulation specific journals (e.g., *Simulation in Healthcare*, *Advances in Simulation*, *International Journal of Healthcare Simulation*). There are also healthcare education journals that publish simulation research (e.g., *Medical Teacher*, *Medical Education*, *Journal of Nursing Education*), and speciality journals may publish simulation research – particularly research through simulation type studies. You should be very wary of 'predatory journals' that solicit for articles. An unsolicited email with 'Dear eminent researcher' should raise your suspicions. Unless you are submitting to a new journal, it is important that the journal is listed on the main search engines (e.g., PUBMED, EMBSCO). You want to ensure that potential readers are able to find your manuscript.

The process of preparing, and submitting, a manuscript is time-consuming. Therefore, it is important to give careful consideration to which journal to submit your manuscript to, and choose a journal where you think you will have a good chance of the paper being accepted, rather than being too aspirational. A useful approach to guiding this decision is to review the reference list of your manuscript. If there is a particular journal that is commonly referenced, then it might be worth considering sending your manuscript to this journal.

In the past, authors were very focused on the impact factor of journals in helping them to decide where to submit a paper. To illustrate, the current impact factor of *Simulation in Healthcare* is 2.7. This means that, on average, every article is referenced 2.7 times. However, this is arguably less important now than in the past as today it is possible to see exactly how many times a particular article is referenced through search engines such as *Google Scholar*. Therefore, we recommend targeting a journal that you think has a readership that would be interested in your article, rather than only focusing on impact factor. If people with an interest in your article are reading it, then hopefully they will also cite it in their own work.

SUBMITTING YOUR MANUSCRIPT

It is very important that you follow the instructions provided by the journal to ensure it is consistent with the style required by the journal – playing particular attention to any word count requirements. You should also write a one-page cover letter to the editor, explaining why you believe your manuscript should be published in the journal. For example, "We believe this study offers a useful contribution to the research. It empirically demonstrates that the generalisation of learning from one medical device to another is not certain and must be explicitly considered and addressed." It is up to the editor to decide whether or not to send out your manuscript for review. So, your letter needs to be succinct and 'sell' your article to the editor.

Once a paper is submitted, you should forget about it for a while. If the manuscript is sent out for review, it may be several months before you receive the reviews and decision. Also, it is important that you only submit your manuscript to one journal at a time.

RESPONDING TO REVIEWER COMMENTS

If your paper does not receive a bench reject (this is where the editor decides not to send the paper out for review), you should eventually receive at least two or three reviews of your manuscript, and a decision by the editor. The decision will be either reject, accept, or revise and resubmit. It is extremely rare to receive an acceptance on first submission to a reputable journal. If your manuscript is rejected, you should read the reviewers' comments, share them with your co-authors, and consider making changes to the manuscript based upon the feedback prior to resubmitting the manuscript to another journal. If you receive a determination of revise and resubmit, you will need to revise your manuscript, detail the changes you have made, and provide a response to every comment from the reviewers.

The comment made by the reviewers may be relatively straightforward to address – for example, "How did you randomise the participants into the two groups?" However, sometimes the comments may require more careful consideration. To illustrate "I disagree with your reasoning for using novice learners who are exposed and fluent in performing only one single method of peripheral intravenous catheterisation to test an untrained device and then drawing conclusions." Either way, it is important to respond to every comment. The easiest way to do this is to prepare a document in which you state each comment, and then provide a response. It may be that you disagree with a particular comment, and elect not to make a change to the manuscript. If this is the case, then you will need to provide a strong justification as to why you did not make the change. Also, if you decide not to make many of the suggested changes (particularly those highlighted by the editor) it may be that your manuscript will be rejected as a result. It is also important to remember that the comments are designed to improve your manuscript – even if it does not feel that way at the time.

Once you have revised your manuscript, and prepared a response to the comments, you should make sure all of the authors agree with the changes, proof-read, and return to the journal. Depending on the extent of the revisions, it may be sent back out to the reviewers, who then may come back with a new set of comments to address. However, hopefully, it will eventually be accepted by the journal.

OTHER FORUMS FOR SHARING SIMULATION RESEARCH

Publication is obviously not the only forum for sharing your research. All of the large simulation societies hold annual conferences, and there are many other national and international simulation, education, and specialty conferences where you can potentially share your research. You may also wish to share your findings at a dissemination event in your institution. This experience can be very valuable in building interest in simulation research and letting people in your organisation know what is happening in your simulation facility. In fact, you may wish to present it at a conference in order to get some feedback on your research before writing it up as a journal article. A conference presentation can be a very good way of getting started with the dissemination of your research activities.

CONCLUSION

There is a growing body of research on healthcare simulation – utilising a range of approaches and methodologies. Most simulation centres have been established in order to provide education and training. This means that these centres may have limited resources to carry out research about simulation. However, healthcare simulation is an under-used tool that has enormous potential to also support the improvement of patient care by research through simulation.

FURTHER READING

Cheng, A., Kessler, D., Mackinnon, R. et al. (2016). Reporting guidelines for health care simulation research: extensions to the CONSORT and STROBE statements. *Advances in Simulation, 1*(1), 1–13.

Cleland, J., Durning, S. J. (2015). *Researching Medical Education.* Oxford: John Wiley & Sons.

Dixon, N. (2001). Writing for publication–a guide for new authors. *International Journal for Quality in Health Care, 13*(5), 417–421.

Howitt, D., Cramer, D. (2007). *Introduction to Research Methods in Psychology.* London: Pearson Education.

Mensh, B., Kording, K. (2017). Ten simple rules for structuring papers. *PLoS Computational Biology, 13*(9), e1005619.

Nestel, D., Hui, J., Kunkler, K., Scerbo, M. W., Calhoun, A. W. (Eds.). (2019). *Healthcare Simulation Research a Practical Guide.* Cham, Swizerland: Springer.

ONLINE RESOURCES

* Equator network – a very good source of reporting guidelines for different types of research studies. See: www.equator-network.org.

REFERENCES

Anton, N., Calhoun, A. C., Stefanidis, D. (2022). Current research priorities in healthcare simulation: results of a Delphi survey. *Simulation in Healthcare, 17*(1), e1–e7.

Bhattacherjee, A. (2012). *Social Science Research: Principles, Methods, and Practices.* Miami, FL: University of South Florida.

Cheng, A., Kessler, D., Mackinnon, R., Chang, T.P., Nadkarni, V.M., Hunt, E.A., Duval-Arnould, J., Lin, Y., Cook, D.A., Pusic, M., & Hui, J. (2016). Reporting guidelines for health care simulation research: extensions to the CONSORT and STROBE statements. *Advances in Simulation, 1*(1), 1–13.

Cleland, J., Durning, S. J. (2015). *Researching Medical Education.* Oxford, UK: John Wiley & Sons.

Gabriel, G., Ramallo, M. A., Cervantes, E. (2016). Workload perception in drone flight training simulators. *Computers in Human Behavior, 64,* 449–454.

Hayden, J. K., Smiley, R. A., Alexander, M., Kardong-Edgren, S., Jeffries, P. R. (2014). The NCSBN national simulation study: a longitudinal, randomized, controlled study replacing clinical hours with simulation in prelicensure nursing education. *Journal of Nursing Regulation, 5*(2), S3–S40.

Howitt, D., Cramer, D. (2020). *Introduction to Research Methods in Psychology.* London: Pearson Education.

Hulley, S., Cummings, S., Browne, r. W., Grady, D., Newman, T. (2009). *Designing Clinical Research,* 4th ed. Philadelphia, PA: Lippincott, Williams & Wilkins.

International Committee of Medical Journal Editors. (2021). Recommendations for the Conduct, Reporting, Editing, and Publication of Scholarly Work in Medical Journals. Available from: www.icmje.org/icmje-recommendations.pdf

Lamé, G., Dixon-Woods, M. (2020). Using clinical simulation to study how to improve quality and safety in healthcare. *BMJ Simulation and Technology Enhanced Learning, 6*(2), 87–94.

McGaghie, W. C., Issenberg, S. B., Petrusa, E. R., Scalese, R. J. (2010). A critical review of simulation-based medical education research: 2003–2009. *Medical Education, 44*(1), 50–63.

Morris, T., Miller, J. C. (1996). Electrooculographic and performance indices of fatigue during simulated flight. *Biological Psychology, 42*(3), 343–360.

Mullin, S., Lydon, S., O'Connor, P. (2020). The effect of operator position on the quality of chest compressions delivered in a simulated ambulance. *Prehospital and Disaster Medicine, 35*(1), 55–60.

Nestel, D., Hui, J., Kunkler, K., Scerbo, M. W., Calhoun, A. W. (Eds.). (2019). *Healthcare Simulation Research a Practical Guide.* Cham, Swizerland: Springer.

O'Connor, P. (2020). ASPiH Conference 2019 keynote paper. Quality improvement through simulation: a missed opportunity? *BMJ Simulation & Technology Enhanced Learning, 6*(4), 193–195.

Qayumi, K., Pachev, G., Zheng, B., Ziv, A., Koval, V., Badiei, S., Cheng, A. (2014). Status of simulation in health care education: an international survey. *Advances in Medical Education and Practice, 5,* 457–468.

Riesenberg, D., Lundberg, G. D. (1990). The order of authorship: who's on first? *Journal of the American Medical Association, 264*(14), 1857.

Stone, P. (2002). Deciding upon and refining a research question. *Palliative Medicine, 16*(3), 265–267.

Walsh, C., Lydon, S., Byrne, D., Madden, C., Fox, S., O'Connor, P. (2018). The 100 most cited articles on healthcare simulation: a bibliometric review. *Simululation in Healthcare, 13*(3), 211–220.

Zheng, Y., Lu, Y., Yang, Z., Fu, S. (2014). Expertise and responsibility effects on pilots' reactions to flight deck alerts in a simulator. *Aviation, Space, and Environmental Medicine, 85*(11), 1100–1105.

11 The Use of Simulation for Quality Improvement

KEY POINTS

- Although there are similarities, quality improvement and research are not the same.
- Healthcare simulation is underutilised as a tool to support quality improvement activities.
- Integrating simulation within quality improvement supports the development of novel quality and safety interventions.
- Using simulation to support quality improvement can address issues for which it may be unethical or impracticable to address using other approaches.

INTRODUCTION

Evidence of poor care experiences and patient harm have prompted the growth of quality improvement (QI) initiatives in recent years (Kaplan et al., 2010). The Academy of Medical Royal Colleges (2016) states that the purpose of QI is to make a difference to patients by improving safety, effectiveness, and experience of care through improved understanding of the healthcare environment. This improvement is achieved by applying a systematic approach to designing, testing, and implementing changes using real-time measurement of improvement. Although the use of simulation for QI is common in other industries (e.g. aviation), the same is not the case in healthcare – yet. There are great opportunities for simulation to make meaningful contribution to patient safety by utilising simulation methods to support QI initiatives.

CHAPTER OVERVIEW

This chapter will:

- provide definitions of QI and translational simulation;
- describe the difference between QI and research;
- identify how simulation can be used to support QI activities and evaluate a range of performance-shaping factors that impact patient safety and quality of care;
- identify how simulation can be used to support adverse event investigations;
- describe a commonly used approach to designing and conducting QI intervention studies; and
- identify reporting guidelines for QI studies.

QI AND RESEARCH

There is sometimes some confusion about the difference between QI and research. This is understandable as there are some similarities between these two activities (O'Connor, 2020). Both activities involve utilising a systematic and structured approach to identifying a problem, collect data,

DOI: 10.1201/9781003296942-11

implement a solution, and test the results. Both activities seek to improve outcomes and there is some overlap between the methods that are used. However, there are a number of important differences between QI and research. These differences are summarised in Table 11.1. Backhouse and Ogunlayi (2020) provide an excellent overview of the similarities between QI and research, as well as other methodologies such as clinical audit and service evaluation.

TABLE 11.1

Differences between QI and Research

Quality Improvement	Research
• Goal is to improve processes and outcomes in a specific unit or setting.	• Goal is to generate generalisable knowledge.
• Aims to understand what works best in a particular clinical context.	• Aims to control extraneous variables that may impact outcomes.
• A criterion of 'good enough' is often applied to data collection and analysis.	• Requires rigour in data collection and analysis.
• Ethical review and approval are not generally required.	• Ethical review and approval are required.
• Findings can generally be adopted immediately in a particular unit.	• There is often a time lag between completing research and adoption of findings.

USE OF TRANSLATIONAL SIMULATION FOR QI

As discussed in earlier chapters, in the past, the main focus of simulation in healthcare has been on education and training. However, simulation can also be a very powerful tool to support organisational learning and improvement (Brazil et al., 2023; Pucher et al., 2017). For example, simulation can be used for testing equipment, processes and systems; it can be used to identify latent threats within a system or for investigating adverse events. These types of activities fit very well with the goals of many QI initiatives. Brazil (2017) proposes the term *translational simulation* as an appropriate term for describing simulation activities that are directly focused on improving healthcare processes and outcomes. The concept of translational simulation lends itself particularly well to QI because of this shared focus. In fact, Brazil (2017) suggests that translational simulation activities will be enhanced if it 'joins the conversation' with quality improvement practitioners and scholars. Translational simulation for QI can be broadly divided into simulation for diagnosis, and simulation for improvement.

SIMULATION FOR DIAGNOSIS

Simulation can be used diagnostically to identify, or investigate, a range of performance-shaping factors that may be challenging to investigate in the actual clinical settings due to practical constraints or ethical concerns (Damschroder et al., 2009). For example, simulation can be used to test a prototype medical device. This is obviously preferable to testing in the real clinical setting. Similarly, simulation can be used to 'diagnose' the impact of fatigue on performance. Again, it is preferable to do this in a simulated environment, rather than the real-world setting.

Performance-shaping factors include a wide range of factors or elements that have been shown to impact human performance in a task, job, or domain (Vincent et al., 1998). Performance-shaping factors can be broadly divided into individual, team, technology, work environment, and system factors (LeBlanc et al., 2011). Each of these factors is discussed below.

INDIVIDUAL FACTORS

Every healthcare worker has a unique set of knowledge, skills, attitudes, and experiences. These factors all impact the delivery of care. Examples of individual performance-shaping factors include:

- demographic factors – age, gender, ethnicity, socioeconomic status, cultural, nationality, language factors;
- cognitive factors – memory, attention, vigilance, reaction time, information processing, problem solving, and error propensity, recognition, and recovery;
- psychological factors – motivation, mood, stress, burnout, fatigue, sleep deprivation, boredom, circadian effects;
- physical attributes – sensory and perceptual (e.g., vision, hearing, tactile ability), anthropometrical (e.g. body size, reach), biomechanical attributes (e.g. strength, force, speed);
- personal attributes – innate personality states or traits;
- preferences and expectations; and
- experience and expertise – knowledge, skills, attitudes, and behaviours.

(LeBlanc et al., 2011)

By way of illustration, simulation provides a safe environment for addressing individual performance-shaping factors on issues such as fatigue (see Example 11.1).

EXAMPLE 11.1   ASSESSING THE EFFECTS OF DIFFERENT WORK SCHEDULES ON CLINICAL PERFORMANCE

The purpose of the study was to assess the effect of different shift patterns on the clinical performance of junior doctors (Gordon et al., 2010). A total of 25 interns participated in the study. The participants were assessed on their management of simulated critically ill patients when rested and after working a traditional shift (24- to 30-hour extended on-call shift) or a modified shift (maximum of 16 scheduled hours). It was found that the junior doctors performed significantly better after working a modified shift as compared to a traditional extended shift. The study authors concluded that the simulation study confirmed the detrimental effect of extended working on clinical performance, and supports the use of simulation as a clinical performance assessment methodology (Gordon et al., 2010).

TEAM FACTORS

Effective teamwork between healthcare workers is crucial to the delivery of high-quality and safe healthcare. Poor teamwork is related to adverse patient outcomes such as the patient morbidity, mortality, and complications, and also to process outcomes such as timeliness of care, error rates, and length of stay (Schmutz & Manser, 2013). Effective teamwork has also been found to support job satisfaction and well-being of healthcare workers (Chang et al., 2009; Rosen et al., 2018). Examples of team performance-shaping factors that can be readily explored through simulation include:

- interpersonal communication – verbal, non-verbal (see Example 11.2);
- teamwork skills and capabilities – leadership/followership, resource allocation, situation awareness, coordination;
- teamwork competences/processes – conflict and conflict resolution, team workload and cognition, task management; and
- team composition – culture, gender, expertise, experience, professions, hierarchy.

(LeBlanc et al., 2011)

EXAMPLE 11.2   IMPACT OF WEARING PERSONAL PROTECTIVE EQUIPMENT (PPE) ON COMMUNICATION

This study examined the effect of wearing PPE on communication between healthcare staff (Hampton et al., 2020). Background noise conditions were simulated from a variety of hospital environments. The participants' ability to interpret speech was assessed both with and without PPE, and with both normal speech and raised voice. Wearing PPE to protect from facial aerosol-generating procedures reduced staff understanding and conventional communication in simulated intensive care unit and operating theatre settings. Loud background environments produced the most pronounced (statistically significant) effect on speech comprehension. There is a need to encourage healthcare staff to speak up, and possibly look for a technological solution to the problem (Hampton et al., 2020).

TECHNOLOGY FACTORS

Technology is an integral part of the delivery of healthcare. The design of technology, and the consideration of the user perspective, are crucial in reducing the likelihood of error. Examples of technology-related performance-shaping factors that can be evaluated through simulation include:

- usability – ease of learning, ease of remembering, ease of use;
- aesthetics, satisfaction;
- anthropometry and biomechanics – posture, grip span, and activation strength requirements;
- flexibility, adjustability, and adaptability;
- component or system failures;
- technology interactions – interfaces, connectivity, communication, and feedback;
- assistance with use before (e.g., training) and during use (e.g., labelling);
- ease of cleaning, upgrades, maintenance, and repair processes and effectiveness;
- version conflicts; and
- obsolescence.

(LeBlanc et al., 2011)

Healthcare workers interface with a wide range of technology – some of which may have error-provoking designs (see Example 11.3). In the USA from 2005 to 2009, a total of 56,000 adverse drug events were associated with the use of infusion pumps. Many of these errors were attributed to issues with the design of the user interface (US Food and Drug Administration, 2010). Recent European and US medical device regulations address the need for usability testing. This regulation reflects the recognition for the need for more effective, safer, and easier-to-use medical devices (European Parliament, 2017).

There is great potential for flaws in the design of technology. These flaws may relate to the design of controls (as in Example 11.3), or with visual or auditory displays (see Example 11.4). Technology, particularly medical devices, should be evaluated in a simulation environment prior to deployment in an actual clinical setting. It is also important that frontline healthcare workers are involved in this evaluation and should be part of the decision- making process about which device(s) to purchase. Simulation should also be used to support the development of medical devices (see Example 11.5).

EXAMPLE 11.3   ERROR-PROVOKING DESIGN

- A doctor set an oxygen flow on the control knob to between 1 and 2 litres per minute for an infant patient.
- The doctor did not know the scale numbers represented discrete, as opposed to a continuous, setting and, in fact, no oxygen flows *between* the settings. The knob rotated smoothly and did not 'click' into place – suggesting that intermediate settings were possible.
- The infant patient became hypoxic before the error was discovered.

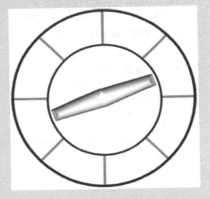

Source: Adapted from Sawyer & CDRH Work Group, 1996

EXAMPLE 11.4   ANAESTHETIC MACHINE ALARM ISSUES

Although alarms are supposed to improve patient safety, a number of problems with alarms in healthcare have been identified. In this study, 10 pairs of trainee anaesthetists participated in a high-fidelity simulation. Unknown to the participants, the oxygen and nitrous oxide pipelines to the anaesthetic machine had been deliberately switched as part of the study. It was found that only 3 out of 10 of the pairs of trainees noticed the transient high nitrous oxide alarm. Although nine of the pairs noticed the low oxygen alarm, this alarm was so loud and distracting that it was muted – perhaps leading the trainees to 'forget' the problem (Mudumbai et al., 2010).

EXAMPLE 11.5   USE OF SIMULATION TO SUPPORT THE DEVELOPMENT OF A PAEDIATRIC INTUBATION AEROSOL CONTAINMENT SYSTEM

In this study, simulation was used to support the development of a paediatric intubation aerosol containment system (IACS) in order to protect healthcare workers from aerosol and droplet generation during intubation (Colman et al., 2021). Five different IACS prototypes were assessed, and feedback was sought from 15 healthcare workers who used the prototypes in simulated clinical scenarios. Failure Modes and Effects Analysis (FMEA; a systematic approach used to identify where failures were likely to occur, and also the relative impact) was also used to identify flaws in the design of the system (known as latent conditions). A total of 32 latent conditions were identified, resulting in five iterations in the development of the IACS prototype. This approach was found to be effective in supporting the user-centred design of a paediatric IACS that reduced the risk to healthcare workers from aerosols generated by intubation (Colman et al., 2021).

WORK ENVIRONMENT FACTORS

Work environment performance-shaping factors are those factors inherent to the design of the work-space or the organisation that affect performance. Examples of work environment performance-shaping factors include:

- interruptions (e.g. alarms);
- distractions (e.g. noise);
- temperature and humidity;
- airflow and venting;
- vibration;
- lighting;
- physical ergonomics of the workspace; and
- space.

(LeBlanc et al., 2011)

Work environment factors have been associated with worker error, fatigue, and discomfort; simulation can be used to identify these factors in the work environment and also to help to identify and test solutions for them in existing workspaces. However, increasingly simulation is also being used more proactively to identify issues in newly constructed healthcare facilities (see Example 11.6).

EXAMPLE 11.6   USE OF SIMULATION TO IDENTIFY SAFETY THREATS IN A NEWLY CONSTRUCTED HEALTHCARE FACILIT

In this study, simulation was used to identify safety threats in a newly constructed paediatric outpatient unit prior to its opening (Colman et al., 2019). Over a three-month period, 31 in situ simulation scenarios were completed, involving 150 participants and 151 observers. This assessment led to the identification of 334 safety issues. A total of 36 of these issues presented a high likelihood for patient harm (e.g. lack of hand hygiene equipment in exam rooms, lack of mechanism to notify the healthcare team of an emergency, no PPE outside exam rooms). The simulations provided a proactive method to identify and mitigate safety issues before the facility received any 'real' patients (Colman et al., 2019).

SYSTEMS FACTORS

Simulation can be used to model and understand systems-level issues. Examples of systems performance-shaping factors include:

- complexity;
- uncertainty;
- risk;
- information flow – quantity and pacing;
- workflow;
- task demands/workload;
- work schedule;
- contextual changes – deviations from what is normal or expected;
- organisational culture and climate;
- policies and procedures;
- incentives and disincentives; and
- pressure for production.

(LeBlanc et al., 2011)

Oftentimes the types of simulation used to assess system factors are computer simulations and models, as opposed to the types of healthcare simulation described in this book. This is sometimes called in silico simulation (Lioce et al., 2020). Examples of in silico simulation include computer-based modelling and utilising simulation to consider different approaches to reducing waiting times (Corsini et al., 2022), or other aspects of workflow in a healthcare unit or hospital (Yousefli et al., 2020). This type of simulation is common in disciplines such as operations research or systems engineering. However, there is also a role for healthcare simulationists to evaluate systems factors using the types of simulation that have previously been discussed in this book. It is important to note that, to bring about change at a systems level, there may be a need to consider individual, team, technological, *and* systems-level performance factors. At the beginning of the COVID-19 pandemic, simulation was widely used to test the preparedness of healthcare facilities to manage COVID-19 patients from a systems perspective (see Example 11.7).

EXAMPLE 11.7   COVID-19 OUTBREAK RESPONSE FOR AN EMERGENCY DEPARTMENT USING IN SITU SIMULATION

This study used in situ simulation to identify system errors and latent safety hazards to prepare for an expected COVID-19 surge (Jee et al., 2020). A series of multidisciplinary, in situ simulations were conducted to identify potential operational errors and latent hazards. Following the simulations, discussions were held with the 39 participants in order to identify where improvements were required in order to improve preparedness. The latent safety hazards identified included narrow hallways, unsuitable clinical spaces, stock issues, and a lack of available protocols to manage a pandemic. Throughout the series of simulations, a steady improvement was also observed in the transfer times from the Emergency Department to the ICU. These improvements were a result of continuous corrective measures based on the analysis of the previous simulation (Jee et al., 2020).

SIMULATION FOR ADVERSE EVENT INVESTIGATION

A particular application of simulation for diagnosis is to support adverse event investigation. It is challenging for healthcare organisations to develop the systems required to investigate adverse events. A rigorous investigation requires individuals with the requisite investigative knowledge and expertise. There is a need to identify the contributing factors to the adverse event – considering all of the performance-shaping factors outlined earlier. Finally, there is a need to develop processes that can be implemented in order to prevent a similar adverse event happening in the future. These are challenges that simulation can help to address. Macrae (2018) outlines five interlinked strategies for how simulation can support adverse even investigation.

- *Support investigator training*. Simulation can be used as an approach for training adverse event investigators. In industries such as aviation, it is common for mishap investigators to conduct simulated investigations using mock wreckage sites, or actors to provide practice in witness interviews or media briefings. In healthcare, past adverse event incident reports could be used for training.
- *Improve investigative infrastructure*. The personnel involved in an adverse event investigation could be assembled in a simulated investigation in order to provide practice for the participants, and to evaluate adverse event investigation protocols.
- *Explore contributory factors and solutions*. Simulation can be used to re-create an adverse event. Such re-creations can provide insights into the performance-shaping factors that contribute to the event and help identify how these issues can be addressed. In the aviation

industry, simulation is commonly used to 're-fly' mishaps in the simulation following an adverse event as part of the mishap investigation (Shy et al., 2002).

- *Embed lessons in practice.* The findings of an adverse event investigation can be used to develop simulation scenarios to train healthcare teams. Again, this is common practice in aviation.
- *Vicariously probe systems.* The findings from an adverse event can be used in other healthcare units in order to test the system, highlight local issues or threats, and identify where processes and work practices need to be improved. The most effective way to carry out such assessments is likely to be through in situ simulation.

SIMULATION FOR IMPROVEMENT

There are many different approaches to conducting a QI intervention to improve the delivery of healthcare. One of the most common approaches to QI is the model for improvement which utilises the plan–do–study–act (PDSA) approach (see Figure 11.1). The four parts of the cycle align with the

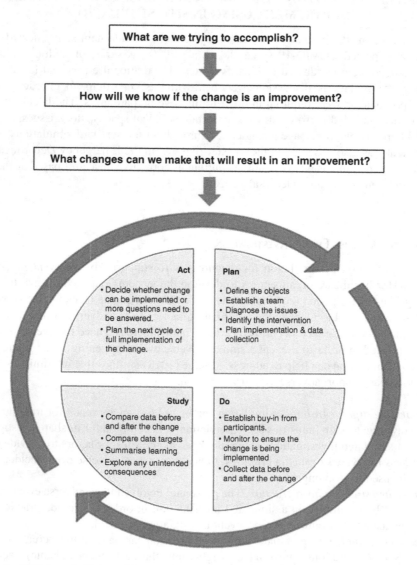

FIGURE 11.1   PDSA cycle (Adapted from ACT Academy NHS Improvement, 2018).

experimental method of developing a hypothesis (plan), implementing an intervention or change to affect an outcome (do), collecting data to test the effects of the change on the outcome (study), and analysing the data in order to make inferences to allow changes to be made to the hypothesis (Taylor et al., 2014). Prior to commencing the PDSA cycle, it is crucial that three questions are answered. These questions are:

1. *What are we trying to accomplish?* There is a need to be very clear on the goal of the improvement process/initiative. Usually, improvement initiatives start with a recognised problem (or problems) within a process that are causing difficulties. This recognition might also be based upon the findings from diagnostic simulation (as discussed above).
2. *How will we know if the change is an improvement?* There is a need identify measure(s) to identify whether the change that we implement to the protocol is actually an improvement.
3. *What changes can we make that will result in improvement?* There is a need to consider what changes we need to make in order to improve the process.

Example 11.8 provides an example of the PDSA approach applied to identify and mitigate latent safety threats in acute airway management. The PDSA approach enables rapid assessment of an intervention, and provides flexibility to make changes rapidly based upon feedback (Taylor et al., 2014).

EXAMPLE 11.8   AN APPLICATION OF PLAN–DO–STUDY–ACT USING SIMULATION

After the first COVID-19 wave, five Emergency Department (ED) staff participated in a PDSA QI study department to improve acute airway management (Yang et al., 2023).

- *Plan.* Surveys and debriefs with ED staff identified emergency airway management as a high-risk procedure that required attention. There were three major categories as areas of potential threats to safety in effective airway management: (1) equipment, (2) infection control, and (3) team communication during acute airway management. An in situ programme was proposed and supported by key stakeholders.
- *Do.* A total of 10 simulations were performed in 2–3 week blocks to identify latent safety threats (LST; defined as errors in design, organisation, training, or maintenance that may contribute to medical errors and have a significant impact on patient safety; Yang et al., 2023). A systems-focused debriefing was carried out after each simulation focusing on the identification of LSTs.
- *Study.* The LSTs identified in the simulations were analysed, and interventions identified to address the LSTs.
- *Act.* The interventions designed to address the LSTs were implemented Emerging LSTs were tracked across each simulation. There was a reduction in the threat associated with LST across the three PDSA cycles that were run.

REPORTING QI STUDIES

Although a study may be considered QI, this does not preclude it from publication. Journals are increasingly interested in publishing QI studies, with some journals specifically focused on publishing QI studies (e.g. *BMJ Open Quality*). However, just as in the case for reporting traditional simulation-based research studies (see Chapter 10), there are also specific reporting guidelines for QI studies called SQUIRE 2.0 (Standards for Quality Improvement Reporting Excellence; Goodman et al., 2016). These guidelines provide useful guidance on what should be reported in a QI study.

CONCLUSION

Healthcare simulation is an under-utilised tool that has great potential in supporting the improvement of patient safety and quality of care through QI. Integrating simulation within QI can support the development of novel quality and safety interventions as well as helping to address issues for which it may be unethical (e.g., evaluate a new medical device) or impracticable (e.g. compare different designs of a new hospital unit) to address using other approaches.

FURTHER READING

Backhouse, A., Ogunlayi, F. (2020). Quality improvement into practice. *British Medical Journal, 368.*

Brazil, V., Purdy, E., Bajaj, K. (2023). *Simulation as an Improvement Technique* (Elements of Improving Quality and Safety in Healthcare). Cambridge: Cambridge University Press. Available from: www.cambridge.org/core/elements/simulation-as-an-improvement-technique/27E6D4C656EAB32476EE582186072551

Institute for Healthcare Improvement: http://www.ihi.org/

O'Connor, P. O'Dea, A. (2021). *An Introduction to Human Factors for Healthcare Workers.* Dublin: Health Services Executive. www.lenus.ie/handle/10147/630666

Revised Standards for Quality Improvement Reporting Excellence, SQUIRE 2.0 http://squire-statement.org/index.cfm?fuseaction=Page.ViewPage&PageID=471

Sawyer, D., CDRH Work Group. (1996). *An Introduction to Human Factors in Medical Devices.* Available from: https://elsmar.com/pdf_files/FDA_files/DOITPDF.PDF

REFERENCES

Academy of Medical Royal Colleges. (2016). *Quality Improvement- Training for Better Outcomes.* London: AMRoC.

ACT Academy NHS Improvement. (2018). *Plan, Do, Study Act (PDSA) Cycles and the Model for Improvement.* Redditch, England: ACT Academy.

Backhouse, A., Ogunlayi, F. (2020). Quality improvement into practice. *British Medical Journal, 368,* m865.

Brazil, V. (2017). Translational simulation, not 'where?' but 'why?' A functional view of in situ simulation. *Advances in Simulation, 2*(1), 1–5.

Brazil, V., Purdy, E., Bajaj, K. (2023). *Simulation as an Improvement Technique.* Cambridge: Cambridge University Press.

Chang, W. Y., Ma, J. C., Chiu, H. T., Lin, K. C., Lee, P. H. (2009). Job satisfaction and perceptions of quality of patient care, collaboration and teamwork in acute care hospitals. *Journal of Advanced Nursing, 65*(9), 1946–1955.

Colman, N., Saldana, C., Craig, K., Edwards, N., McGough, J., Mason, C., Hebbar, K. B. (2021). Simulation-based user-centered design, an approach to device development during COVID-19. *Pediatric Quality & Safety, 6*(4), e47.

Colman, N., Stone, K., Arnold, J., Doughty, C., Reid, J., Younker, S., Hebbar, K. B. (2019). Prevent safety threats in new construction through integration of simulation and FMEA. *Pediatric Quality & Safety, 4*(4), e189.

Corsini, R. R., Costa, A., Fichera, S., Pluchino, A. (2022). A configurable computer simulation model for reducing patient waiting time in oncology departments. *Health Systems.* DOI: 10.1080/20476965.2022.2030655.

Damschroder, L. J., Aron, D. C., Keith, R. E., Kirsh, S. R., Alexander, J. A., Lowery, J. C. (2009). Fostering implementation of health services research findings into practice: a consolidated framework for advancing implementation science. *Implementation Science, 4*(1), 1–15.

European Parliament. (2017). *Regulation (EU) 2017/745 of the European Parliament and of the Council of 5 April 2017 on Medical Devices.* Brussels: Author.

Goodman, D., Ogrinc, G., Davies, L., Baker, G. R., Barnsteiner, J., Foster, T. C., … Kaplan, H. C. (2016). Explanation and elaboration of the SQUIRE (Standards for Quality Improvement Reporting Excellence) Guidelines, V. 2.0: examples of SQUIRE elements in the healthcare improvement literature. *BMJ Quality & Safety, 25*(12), e7.

Gordon, J. A., Alexander, E. K., Lockley, S. W., Flynn-Evans, E., Venkatan, S. K., Landrigan, C. P., Czeisler, C. A. (2010). Does simulator-based clinical performance correlate with actual hospital behavior? The effect of extended work hours on patient care provided by medical interns. *Academic Medicine, 85*(10), 1583–1588.

Hampton, T., Crunkhorn, R., Lowe, N., Bhat, J., Hogg, E., Afifi, W., … Krishnan, M. (2020). The negative impact of wearing personal protective equipment on communication during coronavirus disease 2019. *Journal of Laryngology & Otology, 134*(7), 577–581.

Jee, M., Khamoudes, D., Brennan, A. M., O'Donnell, J. (2020). COVID-19 outbreak response for an emergency department using in situ simulation. *Cureus, 12*(4), e7876.

Kaplan, H. C., Brady, P. W., Dritz, M. C., Hooper, D. K., Linam, W. M., Froehle, C. M., Margolis, P. (2010). The influence of context on quality improvement success in health care, a systematic review of the literature. *Milbank Quarterly, 88*(4), 500–559.

LeBlanc, V. R., Manser, T., Weinger, M. B., Musson, D., Kutzin, J., Howard, S. K. (2011). The study of factors affecting human and systems performance in healthcare using simulation. *Simulation in Healthcare, 6*(7), S24–S29.

Lioce, L., Lopreiato, J., Downing, D., Chang, T.P., Robertson, J.M., Anderson, M., Diaz, D.A., & Spain, A.E., & the Terminology and Concepts Working Group (Eds.) (2020). *Healthcare Simulation Dictionary*. Rockville, MD: Agency for Healthcare Research and Quality. Available from: https://www.ssih.org/Dictionary

Macrae, C. (2018). Imitating incidents, how simulation can improve safety investigation and learning from adverse events. *Simulation in Healthcare, 13*(4), 227–232.

Mudumbai, S. C., Fanning, R., Howard, S. K., Davies, M. F., Gaba, D. M. (2010). Use of medical simulation to explore equipment failures and human-machine interactions in anesthesia machine pipeline supply crossover. *Anesthesia & Analgesia, 110*(5), 1292–1296.

O'Connor, P. (2020). ASPiH Conference 2019 keynote paper. Quality improvement through simulation, a missed opportunity? *BMJ Simulation & Technology Enhanced Learning, 6*(4), 193–195.

Pucher, P. H., Tamblyn, R., Boorman, D., Dixon-Woods, M., Donaldson, L., Draycott, T., … Sevdalis, N. (2017). Simulation research to enhance patient safety and outcomes, recommendations of the Simnovate Patient Safety Domain Group. Simulation research to enhance patient safety and outcomes, recommendations of the Simnovate Patient Safety Domain Group. *BMJ Simulation & Technology Enhanced Learning, 7*(3), S3–S7.

Rosen, M. A., DiazGranados, D., Dietz, A. S., Benishek, L. E., Thompson, D., Pronovost, P. J., Weaver, S. J. (2018). Teamwork in healthcare, Key discoveries enabling safer, high-quality care. *American Psychologist, 73*(4), 433–450.

Sawyer, D., CDRH Work Group. (1996). *An Introduction to Human Factors in Medical Devices*. Washington, DC: US Department of Health and Human Services.

Schmutz, J., Manser, T. (2013). Do team processes really have an effect on clinical performance? A systematic literature review. *British Journal of Anaesthesia, 110*(4), 529–544.

Shy, K. S., Hageman, J. J., Le, J. H. (2002). *The Role of Aircraft Simulation in Improving Flight Safety Through Control Training*. Dryden, CA: NASA.

Taylor, M. J., McNicholas, C., Nicolay, C., Darzi, A., Bell, D., Reed, J. E. (2014). Systematic review of the application of the plan–do–study–act method to improve quality in healthcare. *BMJ Quality & Safety, 23*(4), 290–298.

US Food and Drug Administration. (2010). *White Paper: Infusion Pump Improvement Initiative*. Washington, DC: Author.

Vincent, C., Taylor-Adams, S., & Stanhope, N. (1998). Framework for analysing risk and safety in clinical medicine. *British Medical Journal, 316*(7138), 1154–1157.

Yang, C. J., Saggar, V., Seneviratne, N., Janzen, A., Ahmed, O., Singh, M., … Jafri, F. N. (2023). In situ simulation as a quality improvement tool to identify and mitigate latent safety threats for emergency department SARS-CoV-2 airway management: a multi-institutional initiative. *The Joint Commission Journal on Quality and Patient Safety*. DOI: 10.1016/j.jcjq.2023.02.005.

Yousefli, Z., Nasiri, F.,Moselhi, O. (2020). Maintenance workflow management in hospitals: an automated multi-agent facility management system. *Journal of Building Engineering, 32*, 101431.

Appendix 1: Team Scenario Development Template

CASE SUMMARY

SPECIALTY:	*E.g., Paediatrics, Endocrinology, Respiratory*
TARGET AUDIENCE:	*Who are the learners? Medical SHOS, Interns, New Graduate Nurses*
OVERALL PURPOSE:	*The main target of the session: to understand the roles of every person in the management of an elderly patient with sepsis, to identify…, to escalate… etc.*
KEYWORDS:	*E.g., Sepsis, Sepsis 6 protocol, elderly, post-op*
LEARNING OBJECTIVES: (at the end of the scenario, the learners should be able to…)	• *Recognise…, Prescribe…, Manage…, etc.* • *Aim to include non-technical skills* • •

SCENE INFORMATION

LOCATION:	*What is the simulated setting? Ward-based, Emergency Department, Theatre. You can add in if this is centre-based or in situ*

PARTICIPANTS PER SCENARIO:	*The number of learners that will take part: 2 interns, 2 medical SHOs, 1 ED nurse etc. The scenario may involve a number of learners entering at different time points if you are catering for a lot of learners or if you want to run a pause–discuss/debrief type of simulation, for example:*
	  – *Learners 1 and 2: History and Examination*
	  – *Handover to learners 3 and 4*
	  – *Learners 3 and 4: Investigations and Management*
	  – *Learners 5 and 6: Discharge of patient in part (2) which is 3 days later*

EXPECTED DURATION OF SCENARIO:	*Usually, 10–20 minutes per group of learners*

INFORMATION FOR FACULTY

EXPECTED DURATION OF DEBRIEF	*Ideally double that of the scenario duration*

	This section explains the running of the simulation for those who are delivering the session or "in on" the scenario. It should highlight any points of importance in the scenario – the patient's presentation and history, how the scenarios will progress, the expected actions of the learners, etc. For example:
SUMMARY PLOT FOR FACILITATORS:	*"This scenario begins with a patient who is day 2 post-op from a removal of a tumour in his colon. The patient is starting to display signs of sepsis including shivering. His vitals indicate a clinical deterioration. He also has a developing pneumonia which causes coughing and shortness of breath.*
	When the Interns enter, they should receive a handover from the nurse who explains that the patient is feeling unwell today, like 'he has the flu'. The interns should examine the patient and take a brief history. Possible sites for this infection are a central line which will appear inflamed, the developing pneumonia and possibly post-op sepsis. The patient has a temperature spike, is breathing fast, had a high heart rate and low BP.
	As the scenario develops the patient will become more unwell. He becomes more confused. Blood results will then return which will confirm an infection.
	The interns should call the surgical/medical registrar and microbiology for advice on appropriate antibiotics. They should administer the sepsis 6.
	The scenario should end as the sepsis 6 has been completed and the interns have called for senior help."

INITIAL PATIENT INFORMATION

PATIENT CHART

Patient Name: Age: Gender: Weight:

Presenting Complaint:

RR: 02 Sat: Fi02:

HR: BP: Temp:

Point of Care Glucose:

GCS: Cap Refill Time: INEWS Score:

Triage note:

Allergies:

Past Medical History: Current Medications:

This section should contain a short script that will orientate the learner to the simulated environment. This section should include who they are in the scenario (their role), where they are going, what day and time it is, who the patient is they are going to see is, what they have presented with and what tests have already been done and what is expected of the learner e.g.:

PARTICIPANT BRIEFING:
(to be read aloud to participants before entering the simulation)

"You are the ED intern. It is 2 p.m. on a Monday and you are being called to the ward to see Francis Murphy, a 58-year-old male who is day 2 post-op for removal of a large tumour in his colon.

He is currently receiving slow fluids and has complained to the nursing staff of feeling unwell and 'flu-like' since this morning.

All necessary notes are at the patient's bedside and nursing staff will be available to assist you if needed.

You are to review the patient, conduct a focused history and examination and then formulate a differential diagnosis for the patient's complaints. You are to manage the situation as it develops."

FURTHER PATIENT INFORMATION

Include any relevant history not included in triage note above. Indicate what information will only be given to learners if they ask? Who will provide this information (manikin's voice, sim actors, SP, etc.)?

FURTHER HISTORY

PC:
HPC:
PMHx:
PSHx:
Medications and Allergies:
Social Hx:
Family Hx:
ROS:

PHYSICAL EXAMINATION

List any pertinent positive and negative findings

Cardio: Neuro:
Resp: Head & Neck:
Abdo: MSK/skin:
Other:

PATIENT HISTORY
BRIEFING FOR VOICE
OF THE MANIKIN
OPERATOR:

This section should give key points and lines to the person voicing the manikin in the scenario and should aim to include answers to any questions the learners may ask - Name, age, why you are there, a history, e.g.,

"Your name is Francis Murphy, a 58-year-old male who has just had surgery 2 days ago to remove a tumour in part of your bowel.

Today you have begun to feel 'hot and cold' with a cough and shortness of breath developing. You appear anxious as it has been difficult for the last few days. You are upset as you thought you were recovering well post-op but now feel unwell. You feel 'like you have the flu'.

You don't have any chest pain; you are not coughing up anything.

You have no pain in your abdomen, noting that the nurse changed your wound dressing earlier and it looked 'in good shape'.

The consultant said you can get the NG tube out later and that you are passing small amounts of wind.

The nurse tells you that you have a temperature and that she is calling the doctor.

When the doctor arrives, you can tell your history in full but are anxious. You should cough occasionally and state you 'feel hot and cold'.

Eventually you become drowsier and more disoriented as the scenario progresses. You become more confused."

SUPPORTING TEAM OR FACULTY

EMBEDDED PARTICIPANTS (EP)	*This section lists any individual other than the patient, who is "in on" the scenario, i.e., is scripted to provide realism, additional challenges, or additional information for the learner, for example: paramedic, nurse, receptionist, family member, laboratory technician, microbiology on phone, consultant on-call.*
TECHNICIANS	*Number of technicians required to set up/tear down the scenarios and reset in between – usually* • *Simulation technician* • *A/V technician*
EP's HANDOVER TO PARTICIPANTS: (to be told to participants as they enter simulation)	*This section is a script for the embedded participant to handover to the learners when they enter the room, i.e., what the nurse/paramedic/family member will actually say to the learner, e.g:* *"Hello Doctor. This is Mr. Murphy, a 58-year-old male who was admitted for surgical removal of a large descending colonic tumour. He is now day 2 post-op.* *He was doing fine clinically until today when he began complaining of feeling unwell and flu-like. I have noticed he appears to be shivering in his bed quite a lot.* *He has a central line in situ and a stoma bag which is draining normally.* *He also has a urinary catheter which now has 40 mL of concentrated urine in it.* *His observation sheet is here and it looks like he has a temperature. All of his notes are at the bedside table.* *Mr. Murphy also seems somewhat short of breath.* *Can you please review him?"*
KEY POINTS FOR AN EP or PERSON ANSWERING CALL FOR HELP PHONE CALLS:	*This section should contain prompts for anyone answering the phone if a call for help is initiated. This includes what the person on the other end of the phone would ask, e.g.,* *If this is the Microbiology lab: Name, Board number, DOB, is the patient on abx currently, what have they come in with, what is the clinical picture etc.* *If this is the Blood Bank: Name, Board number, DOB, how much blood do you need, have you sent a group and hold/cross-match, do you require any other blood products etc.* *If this is radiology, surgeons, medics etc.* *Would they take this call or direct elsewhere? What would they ask about this patient? Are they available to come and help if asked?*

TECHNICAL/ENVIRONMENTAL REQUIRMENTS

PATIENT (Select all that apply)	☐ Manikin *(specify type and whether infant/child/adult)* ☐ Standardized participant (SP) *(specify demographics of patient)*
PATIENT APPEARANCE	*This section should detail how the manikin will look for the technician setting up the scenario:* *What is the patient's gender, age?* *Are they sitting up/lying down/tripoding?* *Are they wearing own clothes/hospital gown? TED stockings? Dressings?* *Does the manikin require ACF pads/IO leg etc?* *Do they have any IV lines, catheters, drains etc. in situ? Are they on fluids/oxygen/medications?*
SPECIAL EQUIPMENT REQUIRED	*This section should detail any special equipment requirements, e.g.,* • *NIV/Bipap machine* • *Anaesthetics machine* • *Broselow/arrest trolley* • *Spinal board and C-spine collar* • *Falls alert bracelet*
REQUIRED MEDICATIONS	*E.g., Patient's own medications – inhalers, etc.* *Medications required for the scenario = antibiotics, analgesia, dextrose, nebulisers, etc.* *NOTE: if these are real/live medications, please include the number being used and the person responsible for the sign in and sign out of these medications.*
MOULAGE	*Does the patient have any wounds, rashes, burns, redness around lines?* *Is the patient sweating, pale, etc.?*
PAPERWORK AND RESULTS **(ALL MATERIALS TO BE SOURCED AND PROVIDED AT THE END OF THIS DOCUMENT WITH ALL PATIENT IDENTIFIERS REMOVED)**	*List any paperwork that is required and any test results that may need to be provided to the learner. Include the point in the scenario where these materials are made available to the learner. Some examples are given below:* *Available to learners at start of scenario:* • *Blank EWS* • *Blank Drug Kardex* • *Blank Insulin Prescription* • *Adult summary guidelines of GAPP app printed and available* • *BNF* • *ED admission card (blank/complete)* • *GP letter* *Made available throughout the scenario:* • *Blood results* • *CXR* • *ECG* *Available to learners for Part (b):* • *Chart with admission note/perioperative notes/etc.* • *EWS with 3 days of completed obs* • *Drug Kardex with patient's medications prescribed* • *(on request) DKA guideline* • *ALL RESULTS FROM PART A*

TECHNICAL/ENVIRONMENTAL REQUIRMENTS

Made available during Part (b):
- *ABG/VBG results*
- *Blood results*
- *Repeat ECG*
- *Repeat CXR*
- *Etc.*

MONITORS AT CASE ONSET	☐ Patient on monitor with vitals displayed ☐ Patient not yet on monitor

PATIENT REACTIONS AND EXAM	*Include any relevant physical exam findings that require manikin programming or cues from patient.* *(e.g. abnormal breath sounds, moaning when RUQ palpated, etc.) May be helpful to frame in ABCDE format.*

Scenario States, Learner Actions and Triggers

Patient Vitals	Patient Presentation:		Expected Learner Actions & Triggers to Move to Next State	Facilitator Notes
	Affect/behaviours:	**Clinical signs:**	**Expected learner actions e.g**	**Learner actions that lead to a response**
1. Baseline RR: O₂SAT: % FiO2: HR: Rhythm: BP: T: ℃ GCS:	*E.g., in distress, alert, comfortable, shaking, agitated etc.*	*E.g. Bilateral wheeze, no pulse in right foot, murmur, etc.*	• ABCDE examination • History • Request ABG/lab bloods • •	*E.g., when fluids are given, BP increases to X, if morphine is given, patient becomes nauseous* - -
EWS Score:				

Triggers
What is required for progression to next state, e.g., Sepsis 6 protocol is initiated – move to State 2 (this might be an observed learner action or it might be a time limit etc.)
-

	Affect/behaviours:	**Clinical signs:**	**Expected learner actions:**	**Learner actions that lead to a response:**
2. RR: O₂SAT: % FiO2: HR: Rhythm: BP: T: ℃ GCS:			• • • •	- - -
EWS Score:				

Triggers
What is required for progression to next state, e.g., Sepsis 6 protocol is initiated – move to State 3
-

Scenario States, Learner Actions and Triggers

Patient Vitals	Patient Presentation:		Expected Learner Actions & Triggers to Move to Next State	Facilitator Notes
	Affect/behaviours:	Clinical signs:	Expected learner actions:	Learner actions that lead to a response:
3.				
RR:			•	•
O₂SAT: %			•	•
FiO2:			•	•
HR:				•
Rhythm:				
BP:				
T: °C				
GCS:				
EWS Score:				

RESULTS: LABORATORY RESULTS

Hospital Number:	123456
Name	John TEST
Source	Accident & Emergency

Full Blood Count		
White Cell Count	10*9/L	(4–11)
Haemoglobin	g/L	(115–165)
Platelets	10*9/L	(150–500)
RBC	10*12/L	(3.8–5.8)
Haematocrit	ratio	(0.37–0.47)
MCV	fl	(75–100)
MCH	pg	(26–35)
RDW		(11.0–15.0)
Mean Platelet Volume	fl	(7.5–9.0)
WBC Differential		
Neutrophils	10*9/L	(2.0–7.5)
Lymphocytes	10*9/L	(1.5–4.0)
Monocytes	10*9/L	(0.0–1.5)
Eosinophils	10*9/L	(0.04–0.4)
Basophils	10*9/L	(0–0.1)
Coagulation Screen		
Prothrombin time	Seconds	(11.0–14.0)
APTT	Seconds	(23–35)
INR		
Sodium	mmol/L	(133–146)
Potassium	mmol/L	(3.5–5.3)
Urea	mmol/L	(2.5–7.8)
Creatinine	umol/L	(49–90)
eGFR result/1.73m2	mL/min	
Glucose	mmol/l	(3–6)
	Glucose : ref. range applies to fasting samples	
Calcium	mmol/l	(2.10–2.55)
Adjusted Calcium	mmol/l	(2.10–2.55)
Albumin	g/L	(35–50)
Phosphate	mmol/l	(0.80–1.50)
CRP	mg/L	(<5)
Total Bilirubin	umol/L	(<17)
ALP	iu/L	(25–120)
ALT	iu/L	(<40)
Troponin	mcg/L	(<0.10)
TSH	mu/L	(0.30–5.0)

RADIOMETER ABL FLEX 800

Identifications

Patient ID	123456	
Patient Last Name	TEST	
Patient First Name	John	
Sex	M	
Date of Birth	07/12/1943	
FO2 (l)	21%	
T	37.5	
Sample Type	Venous/Arterial/Capillary	
Operator	AMcB	

Blood Gas Values				
↓	pH		[	7.350–7.450]
↓	pCO2	kPa	[	4.70–6.00]
↓	pO2	kPa	[	11.1–14.4]
	HcTc	%		
Oximetry Values				
↑	c Hb	g/L	[	135–175]
↓	F O2Hb	%	[	94.0–98.0]
↓	sO2	%	[	95.0–99.0]
↓	F CO2Hb	%	[	0.5–1.5]
	F HHb	%	[	0.0–1.5]
	F MetHb	%	[	0.0–1.5]
Calculated Values				
	c Base(Ecf)$_c$	mmol/L		
	c HCO3 · (P)$_c$	mmol/L		
Electrolyte Values				
↓	c Na $^+$	mmol/L	[	136–146]
↓	c K $^+$	mmol/L	[	3.4–4.5]
↓	c Cl $^-$	mmol/L	[	98–106]
↓	c Ca $^{2+}$	mmol/L	[	1.15–1.29]
	Anion Gap c	mmol/L	[	]
Metabolite Values				
↓	c Glu	mmol/L	[	3.0–6.0]
↓	c Lac	mmol/L	[	0.5–1.6]
↓	c Crea	umol/L	[	49–90]

Notes

↑	Value(s) above reference range
↓	Value(s) below reference range
c	Calculated value(s)

URINE ANALYSIS RECORD

PATIENT NAME
PATIENT #
DATE/TIME
pH
BLOOD
PROTEIN
LEUCOCYTES
NITRITES
GLUCOSE
KETONES
OPERATOR ID.

RESULTS: ECGS, X-RAYS, ULTRASOUNDS AND PICTURES

Add any additional files required for running the session such as radiology, ECG results etc. Indicate beside each file what it is (e.g., initial blood results, ABG on room air) and at what point it should be made available to learners during the scenarios (e.g., available at beginning, available on request).

DEBRIEFING TIPS

Including the LOs as a reminder here can be helpful.

DEBRIEFING POINTS
OF IMPORTANCE

Including a structured debriefing framework with prompts can be helpful. A suggested script is below for prebriefing and debriefing and they are to be used as guides only. The facilitators must take care to establish and maintain psychological safety.

Supplemental information regarding any relevant pathophysiology, guidelines, or management information that may be reviewed during debriefing should be provided for facilitators to have as a reference.

DEBRIEFING SCRIPT FOR FACILITATORS

Think about the level of your learners and the purpose of the simulation. SimZone Levels (adapted from Roussin and Weinstock [2017]) are a useful way to do this.

SOME KEY REQUIREMENTS

- Establish the Basic Assumption;
- Invite participation and ensure confidentiality;
- Establish a shared mental model by asking participants or observers to review the events with input from facilitator OR orientate the learners to the scenario;
- Ask open-ended questions and use a conversational/educational technique (self-assessment [+D]; advocacy inquiry [DWGJ]; circular questions [ask an observer to comment]).

USE SILENCE

---

1. WELCOME BACK AND ESTABLISH A SHARED MENTAL MODEL

- Thank the simulation participants and ask them how they feel. [We usually give them a clap]
- Limit this to one or two lines. If they begin to go into the scenario and their actions in depth, say:

> *"Yes, thank you. I want to pause there, and we will come back to that/those points shortly..."*

CHOOSE:

- YOU outline briefly what the scenario was about. Limit this to one or two lines. *"That was a scenario about a 75-year-old man who presented to the ED with neutropaenic sepsis who rapidly deteriorated."*

  or
- In **SimZone Level 2–3,** ask the participants in the scenario to go through the events and actions as they witnessed them.
- Listen.
- Ask the occasional open question *"Tell me more." "What do others think?"*

  or
- You may decide to ask the observers (not the participants) to walk through the events.
     "Tell us in your own words what you observed as the events and actions in that scenario from the time of the handover to the end of the scenario."
- Listen.
- Ask the occasional open question *"Tell me more." "What do others think?"*

---

2. USE A CONVERSATIONAL TECHNIQUE TO EXPLORE THE SCENARIO EVENTS AND ACTIONS AND TO FACILITATE THE DISCUSSION

CHOOSE:

- In **SimZone L1** simulation activities you can guide the learners through the steps and explain what to do and how to do it. This is a **directive feedback** approach to guide development. Use learning objectives to do this or use the workbook provided for medical students.
- In **SimZone L2** simulation activities we go on to use **Plus Delta Framework to Debrief**. This encourages learner **self-assessment**.

PLUS:

- **To the participants *"What went well?"***
  - As they go through each item, listen and then explore the actions with them and the whole group. That means you dig down a little deeper into why it happened, encourage reflection and **close the gap** if there is one. *"Tell me more." "Why did that work out well?" "How do you think you achieved that?" "What is important about that?" "Anything else?" "What does the group think about this?"**
  - If something was particularly good, please spend time discussing how it went so well. We call this unpacking positive performance.

DELTA:

- **To the participants "What went not so well or what could you improve up on?"**
  - As they go through each item, listen and then explore the actions with them and the whole group. That means you dig down a little deeper into why it happened, encourage reflection and **close the gap** if there is one. *"Tell me more?" "I wonder why that happened?" "What led up to that?" "Has anyone experienced this in the clinical setting?" "What does the group think about this?" "How can we make changes or improve?"**
  - If something was of concern from a safety perspective, explain why you are concerned about it and dig down into why it happened by asking open questions and listening carefully for the frame before you start to close the gap.
  - A NOTE ON **CLOSING THE GAP**: This is when we identify a gap between what we saw and what is the accepted standard. That may be a knowledge gap or something that happened due to a lack of situation awareness, feelings or past experiences, or the influence of context. So, you have to listen to the learners as to their reasons why things went the way they did (be they good or not so good).

- In **SimZone L3** simulation activities we use facilitation techniques to gain insight and mental models.
- You can use a modified Plus Delta where you use the technique to start the conversation and then you are spending time facilitating discussions and reflections, analysing and closing the gaps as above.

  <u>or</u>
- You can use an **advocacy inquiry** approach where you use advocacy (speaking) and inquiry (curiosity) to establish the learner's frame.

  - You are making observations on things you saw or heard in the simulation and asking open-ended questions* so that you can analyse the activities.
  - You are trying to get to the reasons (frames) why things happen so once you ask the question you must LISTEN to the answer.
  - Identify the frame** and open that up to the group.
  - Discuss and analyse it, dig down into it and open up the conversation with open-ended questions.
  - Apply it to the real world/clinical practice.
  - Using a **circular questions technique** can be useful here to include the whole group and to promote interprofessional collaboration. Ask an observer from the group to comment on an action they observed in the simulation.

3. **SUMMARY AND WRAP UP**
- Leave time for this at the very end.
- Check that the learning outcomes on the board were covered.
- Address anything that you missed.
- Use this time to address knowledge gaps and to teach.
- Ask each member of the group to tell you one thing they learned that they found valuable.
- Distil and summarise the main points.
- Circulate feedback forms.

*SOME OPEN-ENDED QUESTIONS TO HELP YOU:

- *"Tell me more"*
- *"I am curious as to how you see it/I am curious as to how that happened"*
- *"What were you thinking at the time?"*
- *"What's your take on it?/ Can you talk about that?/ What are your thoughts?/ Can you explain more?"*

**SOME FRAMES THAT YOU MAY ENCOUNTER (and examples):

- Assumptions: *"I thought that it had already been done and I didn't check it"*
- Feelings: *"I was overwhelmed as there was so much to do"*
- Knowledge Base (an obvious lack of knowledge)
- Rules: *"I didn't call the anaesthesiologist because they are only to be called by a senior doctor"*
- Goals: *"I knew we had to get through all the steps in the sepsis 6 protocol so I wanted to get that done ASAP"*
- Situation Awareness: *"I didn't notice the falling BP because I was focused on getting the antibiotic prescribed"*

A note on SimZone Levels (adapted from Roussin & Weinstock, 2017):

- **SimZone L1** is used for *undergraduates* to teach specific skills to a certain standard e.g., follow a protocol. These are instructor-led for educational purposes. The simulation may be stopped and re-started (pause–debrief sim) to provide feedback and guidance. **This is called directive feedback**.
- **SimZone L2** is used for *interns* and *non-native* or *partial teams* (teams who do not normally work together). This is for contextualised clinical skill building. There is usually an embedded participant (EP) and the scenarios run uninterrupted. A Plus Delta debriefing framework is the easiest framework to use. **This promotes self-assessment**.
- **SimZone L3** is for team and systems development for *native teams*. There is no EP. Skilled facilitation is required to support interpersonal risk taking, sharing, reflection and we can use a modified Plus Delta, Debriefing with Good Judgement or similar debriefing framework and also facilitated conversational techniques such as **advocacy inquiry, circular questions** or **guided self-assessment against standards**.

PREBRIEFING SCRIPT FOR FACILITATORS

---

1. WELCOME, CLARIFICATION AND INTRODUCTIONS

"*Welcome to* [insert venue]."

- Outline the Course Objectives:

  "*We are here to practice common scenarios in a supportive learning environment.*"
  "*To work as a team and learn from and with each other.*"
  "*The learning outcomes for this session are* [insert brief learning outcomes].*"

- Introduce yourself and your role and simulation experience.
- If the learners are a mixed group, each person introduces themselves and their background.

SimZone L3
For learners who are regulars to simulation and the session is themed (e.g., respiratory or anaesthetic emergencies), you can begin by asking them to speak about a time they were challenged by a case in clinical practice and how they managed it. This is a good warm-up exercise and can improve the interpersonal risk taking. You may decide to share an experience of your own.

---

2. CREATE A SAFE ENVIRONMENT FOR LEARNING AND SHARING [PSYCHOLOGICAL SAFETY]

"*When you come here, we demonstrate respect and curiosity, and we operate a few basic principles:*"

"*We believe that everyone here is INTELLIGENT, CAPABLE, CARES about doing their BEST and wants to IMPROVE.* This is what we call **The Basic Assumption.**"

"*We respect **Confidentiality***. *We are here to learn together, and this is not an assessment or test or something we share with others after the simulation. We are all curious and want to learn more.*"

"*We want everyone to **Participate** and contribute to this learning experience, so we invite you to all jump right into the experience.*"

- IF NECESSARY, clarify **Boundaries** (if any) (e.g., "*the patient will not arrest; the patient will die no matter what you do*", "*there is a challenging part in the scenario where you are expected to speak up*" etc.).

3.   OUTLINE WHAT IS EXPECTED OF THE LEARNERS/STUDENTS

"Each scenario lasts [insert time] *with a* [insert time] *debrief afterwards."*

"We want you to immerse yourselves fully and to do that you have to suspend reality. We have done our best to make this feel real but we can only do so much so we need you to meet us halfway and agree that although this is not real, you will do your best to behave as naturally as you can. This is the **Fiction Contract** *that we make with all learners."*

"We understand that this can be stressful and that is a normal part of simulation and is something that everyone experiences."

"An **embedded participant** *or* **confederate** *may be present in the simulation, and they are there to help you. They will do the following* [insert the outline of things they do e.g., cannulation, ECGs etc.]."

"You will be operating at [insert grade] *level (e.g., your own grade and behave exactly as you normally do, intern, SHO) and you will be orientated to the scenario before you go in (e.g., you will be told the time, situation and what you are being asked to do)."*

"We have some infection control requirements (e.g., you are to wear a mask, visor, clean after you use the stethoscope etc.)."

4.   ORIENTATE THE LEARNERS TO THE SIMULATION SPACE. {THIS IS IMPORTANT FOR HEALTH AND SAFETY}

- Demonstrate and explain:
    - The functionality of the manikin. What it can and cannot do.
    - How the clinical paperwork is presented (e.g., EWS, clinical notes, results). Remind learners to **WRITE IN PENCIL** on all prescriptions, clinical notes etc.
    - How to use any other clinical equipment {defib, infusion pump}, including the phone and how to operate it for escalation of care.
    - Make learners aware of any AV/viewing or recording technology in use.
    - Housekeeping: The location of the toilet, the use of mobile phones etc.

5.   BRIEF THE PARTICIPANTS BEFORE THEY ENTER THE SIMULATION

- See individual case scenario and brief the participants.

    "It is 4 a.m. on a Sunday and you are the SHO on call, the triage nurse etc. You are presented with a 75-year-old male with ...."

Appendix 2: Standardised Participant Case Development Template

This is the template used by the Irish Centre for Applied Patient Safety and Simulation (ICAPSS) for standardised participant scenarios, which was developed by the Association of SP Educators (ASPE). The latest version of the ASPE case development template is available from: www.aspeducators.org/aspe-case-development-template.

In earlier printings of this book we erroneously took credit for the development of this template, instead of attributing it to the actual developers - the ASPE. This is an oversight for which we, the authors, are responsible and for which we apologise.

TABLE OF CONTENTS

Part 1 Overview & Administrative Details

Part 2 – Door Chart/Note & Learner Instruction

Part 3 – Case Content for SPs

Part 4 – Create A Checklist for the SP Case (Examiner and/or SP)

Part 5 – Checklist Guidelines/Anchors

Part 6 – Additional Learner Materials

Part 7 – Post-Encounter Activities/Task

Part 8 – Checklist (Rubric or Answer Key) for Post-Encounter Activities

Part 9 – Prebrief/Learner Orientation (if required)

Part 10 – Debriefing (if planned)

GUIDE TO USING THIS TEMPLATE

This template is intended to be comprehensive in nature but may not contain every element necessary for an activity or scenario. Conversely, not every activity or scenario will require each part of this template. This record should make the reproduction of this SP Encounter/station easy. Each of the sections 'speaks' to a different group so there may be repetition in some content.

NOTE: SP educators/case developers may exercise their judgement when selecting which parts of this template are applicable to their activities or scenarios. Some parts of this template may not be relevant to your case development and these parts of the template can be deleted.

This template contains suggestions and examples which you can delete when populating the information for your case.

Part 1 – Overview & Administrative Details

PATIENT/SP NAME

NAME OF THE CASE/ENCOUNTER, OVERVIEW & EXPECTATIONS FOR THE LEARNER: *(E.G., ITCHY RASH IN A 25-YEAR-OLD. MRS X IS A 25-YEAR-OLD LADY ATTENDING HER GP BECAUSE SHE IS CONCERNED RE AN ITCHY RED RASH ON THE FLEXOR ASPECTS OF HER ARMS & LEGS. THE DIAGNOSIS IS ECZEMA AND THE LEARNER IS EXPECTED TO TAKE A FOCUSED HISTORY, EXAMINE THE RASH & MAKE THE MOST LIKELY DIAGNOSIS)*

PATIENT'S REASON FOR THE VISIT *(E.G., WHY IS THE PATIENT COMING TO THE DOCTOR TODAY?)*

PATIENT'S CHIEF COMPLAINT:

DIFFERENTIAL DIAGNOSIS:

ACTUAL DIAGNOSIS:

CASE PURPOSE OR GOAL: *(E.G., FORMATIVE, SUMMATIVE, TEACHING, LEARNER PRACTICE, ASSESSMENT, LECTURE, DEMONSTRATION)*

LEVEL OF THE LEARNER AND DISCIPLINE: *(E.G., 3RD YEAR NURSING; GP TRAINEE ETC.)*

LEARNER'S
PREREQUISITE
KNOWLEDGE & SKILLS:

LAY SUMMARY OF
PATIENT STORY:

LEARNING/CASE
OBJECTIVES:

LIST OF ASSESSMENT
INSTRUMENTS USED:
(E.G. SP CHECKLIST,
POST-ENCOUNTER NOTE,
QUIZ)

EVENT FORMAT &
DURATION OF THIS &
EACH STATION *(E.G.,*
FORMATIVE, SUMMATIVE
END OF YEAR OSCE,
MULTI STATION OSCE)

DEMOGRAPHICS OF
PATIENT/RECRUITMENT
GUIDELINES: *(E.G.,*
AGE RANGE, GENDER,
BODY TYPE, ETHNICITY,
OTHER)

LIST OF SPECIAL
SUPPLIES NEEDED
FOR ENCOUNTER/
STATION SET UP:
(E.G., ADDITIONAL
MATERIALS (see part 6)
MOULAGE, PROPS, SP
ATTIRE, PHYSICAL EXAM
EQUIPMENT, ETC.)

SP REFERENCE
MATERIALS IF NEEDED:
(E.G., ANY REFERENCES
OR LINKS TO VIDEOS,
IMAGES OR WEBSITES OF
PHYSICAL SIGNS ETC.)

ANY SPECIAL
INSTRUCTIONS FOR
SUPPORT STAFF:
(E.G. SIM TECH, SIM
EDUCATOR, FACULTY)

Part 2 – Door Chart/Note & Learner Instructions

SETTING (PLACE/TIME):

PATIENT NAME:
AGE:
GENDER:
CHIEF COMPLAINT:

VITAL SIGNS: (IF APPLICABLE)
    RESPIRATORY RATE
    OXYGEN SATURATIONS
    HEART RATE
    BLOOD PRESSURE
    TEMPERATURE
    BMI

LAB RESULTS: (IF APPLICABLE)
IMAGE RESULTS: (IF APPLICABLE)

INSTRUCTIONS TO LEARNERS:
- Tasks to be completed (e.g., elicit an appropriate history, conduct a focused physical exam)
- Patient encounter length (10 minutes, 20 minutes, 30 minutes, etc.)

Part 3 – Case Content for SPs

PRESENTATION & RESULTING BEHAVIOURS *(E.G., BODY LANGUAGE, NON-VERBAL COMMUNICATION, VERBAL CHARACTERISTICS)*	**General affect**: e.g., pleasant and cooperative **Body language**: e.g., relaxed **Facial expression**: e.g., relaxed **Eye contact**: e.g., natural If required – note any specific reactions required in specific circumstances e.g., if the learner asks about x then you (SP) will become tearful/agitated/calm etc.
OPENING STATEMENT – THE FIRST THING THAT YOU (SP) SAYS WHEN STUDENT/CANDIDATE COMES IN/SITS DOWN ETC.	
GUIDANCE ON DEALING WITH OPEN-ENDED QUESTIONS AND GUIDELINES FOR DISCLOSURE:	• Information offered spontaneously (what the patient can disclose after an open-ended question) • Information hidden until asked directly (what the patient should withhold until specific questioning)
HISTORY OF PRESENT ILLNESS (HPI):	**Quality/Character**: **Onset**: **Duration**: **Location**: **Radiation**: **Intensity**: **Aggravating Factors (what makes it worse)**: **Alleviating Factors (what makes it better)**: **Precipitating Factors (does anything seem to bring it on?)**: **Associated Symptoms**: **Significance to Patient (impact on patient's life, patient's beliefs about origin of problem, underlying concerns/fears, expectations for the visit)**:
REVIEW OF SYSTEMS: *(E.G., PERTINENT POSITIVES & NEGATIVES)*	

PAST MEDICAL HISTORY (PMHx):	**Illnesses/Injuries:**
	Hospitalisations:
	Surgical History:
	Screening/Preventive (if relevant):
	Medications (prescription, over the counter, supplements):
	Allergies (e.g., environmental, food, medication and reaction)
	Gynecologic History (if relevant):

| **FAMILY MEDICAL HISTORY:** | **Family Tree (e.g., health status, age, cause of death for appropriate family members):** |
| | **Relevant Conditions/Chronic Diseases (management/treatment):** |

SOCIAL HISTORY:	**Substance Use (past and present):** **Drug Use (recreational and medications prescribed to other people):** **Tobacco Use:** **Alcohol Use:**
	Home Environment:
	Social Supports:
	Occupation:
	Relationship Status:
	Current Sexual Partners (if relevant):
	Lifetime Sexual Partners (if relevant):
	Safety in Relationship (if relevant):
	Leisure Activities:
	Diet:
	Exercise:

PHYSICAL EXAM FINDINGS:

PROMPTS & SPECIAL INSTRUCTIONS:	**Questions the patient MUST ask/ statements patient must make (optional)**
	Questions the patient will ask if given the opportunity
	What should the patient expect from this visit?

| GUIDELINES FOR FEEDBACK FOR SP (IF REQUIRED): | (e.g., logistics, content for feedback) |

Part 4 – Create A Checklist for the SP Case (Examiner and/or SP)

LEARNER NAME:	. XXX
DATE:	. XXX
SP CASE NAME:	.
GRADING SCALE (LIKERT OR DICHOTOMOUS):	Please describe the scale to be used for each item in this section (e.g., Yes/No, Done/Not Done, etc.). Include the point values for each (e.g., Yes = 1, No = 0). Insert checklist here (you can insert more than one checklist if the examiner and SP are assessing different things). You may decide that only the examiner is using a checklist. NOTE When creating a checklist, don't forget to create a **Global Rating Scale** also.

Part 5 – Checklist Guidelines/Anchors

Checklist guidelines are a description of the intent of a checklist item. Not all items on a checklist must be included; however, clarification of certain items may be useful for examiners.

This includes specifics of what examiners should be looking for in order to receive credit for an item. Include examples of questions or approaches a student might take and the appropriate response.

Examples below for a history and examination checklist with anchors *(note these are institution-specific; authors do not intend example criteria to serve as recommendations for a specific technique)*

HISTORY CHECKLIST:	Learner asks about shortness of breath: Checklist could be YES or NO **You could add in the following anchors/descriptiors**: *Note to scorers: Any questions about trouble breathing, difficulty breathing or trouble catching breath would warrant credit for this item.* **You could add in the following anchors/descriptors**: Note to scorers: Questions about "lung problems" would not warrant credit for this item.
PHYSICAL EXAMINATION CHECKLIST:	Learner palpated the area of pain. Checklist could be DONE, DONE INCORRECTLY or NOT DONE **You could add in the following anchors/descriptors**: Done: The learner will place his hand OR fingertips right over the area of pain. Done incorrectly: The student does this manoeuvre over gown (or other clothing).

Part 6 – Additional Learner Materials

Attach any required materials to this section *(e.g. laboratory results/readings, images, physical exam results cards)*

Part 7 – Post-Encounter Activities/Task

POST-ENCOUNTER ACTIVITIES/TASK	**Describe in detail the type of activity the student will engage after the SP Encounter.** It might be to write a Subjective, Objective, Assessment and Plan (SOAP) note, request labs and complete the paperwork, perform a procedure (venepuncture), obtain consent or handover to another person or it could be to write a reflection or even to answer multiple choice questions, etc.)

Part 8 – Checklist (Rubric or Answer Key) for Post-Encounter Activities

You can insert your checklist here for the post-encounter task. You can use one that best fits the task described.

Part 9 – Prebrief/Learner Orientation (if required)

FORMAT AND TIMING:	*E.G., This is a high-stakes OSCE station. It lasts 12 minutes. You have 8 minutes for the patient encounter and 4 minutes for a post-encounter task which will be to xxx*
SESSION OBJECTIVES:	*E.G., The purpose of this station/encounter/circuit is to xxx*
SPECIAL INSTRUCTIONS: (E.G., SPECIAL EQUIPMENT)	

Part 10 – Debriefing (if planned)

TECHNIQUE TO BE
USED: (E.G. PLUS-DELTA,
ADVOCACY-INQUIRY,
DEBRIEFING WITH
GOOD JUDGEMENT)

DISCUSSION
QUESTIONS/TOPICS:

Index

Pages in *italics* refer to figures, pages in **bold** refer to tables.

A

abstract conceptualisation, 18, 19, 68
ACLS, 20, 21
active experimentation, 19
ADDIE model, 23–35, *24*
    application, 98
adult learning
    andragogy, 13
    theory, 21
    see also learning theories
advanced cardiac life support, *see* ACLS
Advances in Simulation (journal), 9
advocacy-inquiry, 73; *see also* debriefing
Analyse, Design, Develop, Implement, Evaluate,
    see ADDIE
andragogy, 13; *see also* adult learning; Knowles, Malcolm
anxiety, of learners, 57
ASPE, 47, 56, 61
ASPiH, *see* Association for Simulated Practice in
    Healthcare
assessment
    drives learning, 81
    formative, 82–83
    frameworks, 85–89
    simulation educators, of, 89–90
    summative, 82–83
    value of, 83, 90
Association for Simulated Practice in Healthcare, 8
Australian Society for Simulation in Healthcare, 8
Association of Standardized Patient Educators,
    see ASPE

B

Bandura, Albert, 16–17
behavioural learning
    precision, *see* precision teaching
    task analysis, 16
    theory, 13–16, 21
    see also deliberate practice; learning theories
behavioural markers, 87
behaviourism, 13; *see also* behavioural learning
Bloom's taxonomy, 26, 27, *27*, 36

C

CAVE, 5
Cave Automatic Virtual Environment, *see* CAVE
clinical outcomes, 1, 8
Clinical Simulation in Nursing (journal), 9
cognition, 17; *see also* social cognitive learning theory
competency, healthcare providers, of, 2
computer-based simulators, 5
    modelling, 5
    realism of, 5
    see also virtual reality simulators; in silico
conceptualisation, abstract, *see* abstract conceptualisation
concrete experience, 19
confederate participant, *see* embedded participant
confidentiality, 63
constructive alignment, 81
constructivist learning theory, 18–19, 21
    experiential learning, 18–19
    see also learning theories
cry wolf phenomenon, 52

D

debriefing
    application, 69–75
    conversational, 71
    DASH, 64, 77, **78**, 79, 90
    definition of, 68
    descriptions phase, 70
    difficulties with, 75
    facilitators, 72
    formative assessment, as, 74–75
    importance of, 67
    judgement with, 73
    learning insights from, 67, 69
    learning objectives and, 69
    methods, 69–75
    micro-debriefing, 15
    psychological safety and, 68–69
    reactions, 70
    scripted, 74
    structure, 70
    timing, 72
    video-assisted, 73–74
    see also prebriefing
Debriefing Assessment for Simulation in Healthcare, *see*
    debriefing, DASH; debriefing
deliberate practice, 14–15
    observation vs, 14
    precision teaching and, 16
    rapid cycle, 14
didactic teaching, 15, **77**

E

educational intervention evaluation, *33*, 84, 105
embedded participant, 6, 41, **130**
    simulated participant, distinction from, 4
embedded patient, *see* embedded participant
environmental fidelity, 7; *see also* fidelity
equipment fidelity, 7; *see also* fidelity
Ericsson, K. Anders, 14
    Kolb's theory of, 18, 28, 68
    see also constructivist learning theory; learning theories
ethics, 2, 99
    research, of, 106

evaluation hierarchy, Kirkpatrick's, *see* Kirkpatrick model
experiential learning, 18–19
    cycle of, 18, 68

F

facility, simulation
    accreditation, 99
    ADDIE, 98
    challenges, 92
    education, 97
    equipment sourcing, 95–96
    financing, 95
    management systems, 99
    personnel, 96–97
    planning, 100, **101**
    priorities, **93**
    qualifications, 97
    resources, 95
    staff, 96–97
    training, 97
feedback
    directive, 72
    virtual reality simulators, from, 6
FHSS, 39, 50, 51, 54, **55**, 56
healthcare, 93–94
fidelity, 6–7, **55**, 85, 86
    definition of, 6–7
    dimensions of, three, 7
    high, 7, 12, 119
    low, 7
    medium, 32
    see also realism
Foundation for Healthcare Simulation Safety, *see* FHSS
functional task alignment, 7; *see also* fidelity

G

Gladwell, Malcolm, 14
goals, 63, 75, 84, 100, 116, 142
    learning, in, 6, 14, 16, 63–64
    personal, 18
    setting of, 18, 63, 94
    teacher, of, 18

H

HALO, 3
healthcare providers, *see* providers, of healthcare
healthcare simulation, 1
    acceptance of, 7
    conferences, 8–9
    definition of, 1
    effectiveness, 8
    history of, 1
    journals, 9
    learners, impact on, 8
    manufacturing companies of, 10, 98
    patients, impact on, 8
    societies, 8–9
High Acuity Low Occurrence, 3
HRA, *see* human reliability analysis
human reliability analysis, 16
hybrid simulation, 5; *see also* table-top simulation

I

ICAPSS, 39, 43, 44, 54, 93, 94
imitation, 17
    see also social cognitive learning theory
implementation science, 29
in silico, 5, 121; *see also* computer-based simulators
in situ simulation, 5–6, 48
    table-top simulation, distinction from, 5–6
instructional design
    definition, 23
    evaluation, 30
    implementation, 29
    see also ADDIE
International Journal of Healthcare Simulation, 9
International Nursing Association for Clinical Simulation
    and Learning, 8, 9
Introduction, Situation, Background, Assessment,
    Recommendation, *see* ISBAR
Irish Association for Simulation, 8
Irish Centre for Applied Patient Safety and Simulation, *see*
    ICAPSS
ISBAR, 26

J

Journal of Surgical Simulation, 9

K

kinaesthetic learning, *see* learning by doing
Kirkpatrick model, 30–33, 35
Knowles, Malcolm, 13
Kolb, 19
    theory, *see* experiential learning theory

L

learner
    centred, 18, 26, 71
    expectations, 62–64
    experience, 7
    performance, 82
learning
    by doing, 18
    needs, 6, 23, 63, 67, 72, 78
    objectives, 69
    process, 81
learning theories
    adult, 13
    behavioural, *see* behavioural learning theory
    combining of, 14, 19–21
    independent, 13
learning theory, 12
    SBE, absence in design of, 12
life support skills, 3, 20

M

mastery learning, 20–21
McGaghie, 14, 20; *see also* deliberate practice
management systems, simulation, *see* simulation
manikin simulators, 3–4
    functions of, 3

storage of, 4
mannequin, *see* manikin simulators
manufacturing companies, healthcare simulation, of, 10, 98
modelling, 17
    computer-based, 5; *see also* social cognitive learning
        theory
morals, *see* ethics

N

nasogastric tube insertion, 16, **17**, 41
New World Kirkpatrick Model, *see* Kirkpatrick Model
NGT, *see* nasogastric tube insertion
non-technical skills
    assessment of, 86–89
    communication, 86
    leadership, 86
    self-management, 86
    social, 86
    teamwork, *see* teamwork
NWKM, *see* Kirkpatrick model

O

Objective Structured Clinical Examination, *see* OSCE
objectives of learning, 26
observation, 17
    deliberate practice vs, 14
    see also social cognitive learning theory
Observational Structured Assessment of Debriefing Tool,
        see OSAD
OSAD, 76–77
OSCE, 46, **88**
    educational impact, 85
outcomes of learning, 26, 81
oxygen saturation, 3, 43, **148**

P

patient
    assessment, 4
    experiences, 115
    outcomes, 8
Pavlov, Ivan, 13
PDSA, 123
plan, do, study, act, *see* PDSA
plastic person, *see* manikin simulators
Practical Obstetrics Multi-Professional Training package,
        see PROMPT
prebriefing, 62–64; *see also* debriefing
precision teaching, 14, 15–16, 34, 85
    deliberate practice and, 16
    impact of, 34
procedural skills, 6, 14, 20
    assessment of, 85–86
    clinical, 25
programme design, 9
PROMPT, 30
providers, of healthcare
    competencies, 2
    training needs, 2
    see also SBE

psychological fidelity, 7, 85; *see also* fidelity
psychological realism, *see* psychological fidelity, fidelity
psychological safety, 57–58
    death of simulator, 59–60
    debriefing and, 68–69
    deception, 58–59
    hidden agendas, 58
    professional identity, 58
    scenario-based threats, 58
    validity, 58

Q

QI
    individual factors, 117
    research, distinguishing from, **116**
    reporting of, 114
    system factors, 120
    team factors, 117
    technology factors, 118
    translational simulation, 116
    work environment factors, 120
quality improvement, *see* QI

R

rapid cycle deliberate practice, 14
    efficacy of, 15
    see also debriefing; deliberate practice
real person, *see* simulated participants
realism
    computer-based simulators, of, 5
    definition of, 6
    educational impact, 85
    learners and, 58
    limitations of, 58, 64
    simulated participants, in, 4
    simulation and, 2, 6
    virtual reality simulators, of, 5
REAPS, 16
reflection, 67; *see also* debriefing
reflective observation, 19; *see also* debriefing
reflective practice, 68; *see also* debriefing
research
    ethical, 106
    examples, 105, 106
    feasibility, 106
    publication, 107–112
    question, 107
    QI, distinguishing from, **116**
    simulation for, 8, 104–113
Retain, Endure, Adapt, Perform, Stability, *see* REAPS
reward, learning without, 17
risks, 47
    learners, to, 47
    patients, to, 48, 51, 56
    simulated participants, to, 53
    staff, to, 53, 55
    see also safety
role-play, 6
Rudolph's recommendations for learning objectives,
        26–27

S

safety
environment, 61–62
equipment, 51, 53
facilities, 54, 61–62
medication, 49, 51
management of, 50
negative transfer, 52
patients, 48, 51, 56, 119
physical, 47
policies, 53–55
professional guidance, 54
psychological, *see* psychological safety
reporting processes, 55
resource use, 52
simulated participants, 60–61
staff, 55
see also risks
SBE, *see* simulation-based education
scenarios
high-risk, 6
faculty information, 40
information for, 40
modelling of, 5; *see also* computer-based participants
simulation-based education, 38, 46
simulated participant, 43–46
team, 39
writing, 38–39
self-directed learning, 18
self-efficacy, 15, 17–18, 21
self-regulation, 17–18
serious game, 5; *see also* computer-based simulators
SESAM, *see* Society in Europe for Simulation Applied to Medicine
SimGHOSTS, 10, 102
SimZones, 6
simulated participants, 4
case content for, 45
embedded participant, distinction from, 4
feedback for learner from, 45
realism of, 4
simulated patients, *see* simulated participants
simulated task, 14, 19; *see also* rapid cycle deliberate practice
simulation
advantages of, 2–3
definition of, 1
deliberate practice and, 14; *see also* deliberate practice
diagnosis, for, 116
effectiveness of, 7–8
facility, *see* facility, simulation
healthcare, of, *see* healthcare simulation
improvement, for, *122*
limitations, 2
management systems, 99
realism, vs, *see* realism
simulators, distinguishing from, 1
simulation-based education, 2, 68
clinical outcomes and, 8
debriefing, 67

designing of, 7, 12, 13, 49
ethics, 2
evaluation, 101, 104
goal of, 38
impacts of, 8, 67
intervention, 31
learners, expectations of, 13–14
learners, impacts on, 67
reflective practice and, 78
requirements for, 92
scenarios and, 38, 46
Simulation in Healthcare, 9
simulators
advantages of, 2–3
computer-based, 5, 121
manikin, *see* manikin simulators
participant-based, *see* simulated participants
simulation, distinguishing from, 1
table-top, 5; *see also* table-top simulation
task trainer, 1, 4, 5, 19, 83
virtual reality, 5, 6, 102
skills
non-technical, *see* non-technical skills
transference, 3
social cognitive learning theory, 16–19, 21; *see also* learning theories
Society in Europe for Simulation Applied to Medicine, 9, 99; *see also Advances in Simulation*
Society for Simulation in Healthcare, *see* SSH
Society of Surgical Simulation, 8
SP, *see* simulated participants
SPLINTS, 88–89
SSH, 3, 8, 35, 54, 98–100, 102
standardised patients, *see* simulated participants
Surgical Simulation, Society of, 8

T

table-top simulation
realism of, 5
in situ simulation, distinction from, 5–6
task trainer, 4
teacher-centred, 26
teamwork, 4, *24*, 48, 72, 76, 86
theory, definition of, 12
training
effect, isolation of, 32
ideas for, 25
piloting, 29

V

VAD, *see* debriefing, video assisted
venepuncture, 3, 14, 15, **86, 154**
video-assisted debriefing, *see* debriefing
virtual patient, 5
virtual reality simulators, 5
feedback from, 6
realism of, 5
see also computer-based simulators

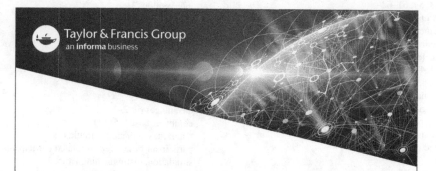

Printed in the United States
by Baker & Taylor Publisher Services